CLARE BAMBRA, LUKE MUNFORD,
SAM KHAVANDI, AND NATALIE BENNETT

WITH A FOREWORD BY
HANNAH DAVIES AND SÉAMUS O'NEILL

NORTHERN
EXPOSURE

COVID-19 and Regional Inequalities
in Health and Wealth

POLICY PRESS SHORTS RESEARCH

First published in Great Britain in 2023 by

Policy Press, an imprint of
Bristol University Press
University of Bristol
1–9 Old Park Hill
Bristol
BS2 8BB
UK
t: +44 (0)117 374 6645
e: bup-info@bristol.ac.uk

Details of international sales and distribution partners are available at
policy.bristoluniversitypress.co.uk

British Library Cataloguing in Publication Data
A catalogue record for this book is available from the British Library

ISBN 978-1-4473-6922-6 hardcover
ISBN 978-1-4473-6924-0 ePub
ISBN 978-1-4473-6923-3 ePdf

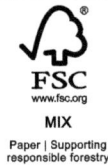

Contents

List of figures and tables

Figures

Tables

List of abbreviations

CCG	Clinical Commissioning Group
COPD	Chronic Obstructive Pulmonary Disease
GDP	Gross Domestic Product
GHQ-12	General Health Questionnaire 12
GVA	Gross Value Added
IMD	Index of Multiple Deprivation
IMR	Infant Mortality Rate
LAD	Local Authority District
LSOA	Lower Super Output Area
MSOA	Middle Super Output Area
NCD	Non-Communicable Diseases
NHS	National Health Service
ONS	Office for National Statistics
SES	Socio-Economic Status
UKHLS	UK Household Longitudinal Study (or Understanding Society)

About the authors

Clare Bambra is Professor of Public Health at the Population Health Sciences Institute, Newcastle University. She is an interdisciplinary social scientist working at the interface of public health, health politics and policy, health geography and social epidemiology. Twitter @ProfBambra

Natalie Bennett is a research associate in the Population Health Sciences Institute at Newcastle University working on health inequalities. She is a Social Epidemiologist with a background in Human Geography and interests in the social determinants of health. Twitter @DrNCBennett

Sam Khavandi is a research associate in Health Economics at the University of Manchester. He is an applied health economist with a background in public health focusing on the wider determinants of health and consequences of health inequalities.

Luke Munford is Senior Lecturer in Health Economics at the University of Manchester. He is an applied economist who applies statistical and econometric techniques to secondary data to understand the causes and consequences of health inequalities. Twitter @dukester24

Acknowledgements

This book is based on a series of policy reports published with the Northern Health Science Alliance (NHSA). We would like to acknowledge Hannah Davies of the NHSA as well as the other colleagues who contributed to the policy reports: Nasima Akhter, Benjamin Barr, Kate Bernard, Tim Doran, Evangelos Kontopantelis, Paul Norman, Kate Pickett, Matt Sutton, David Taylor-Robinson, Sophie Wickham. We gratefully acknowledge the support of our funders: CB and NB are funded by the NIHR Applied Research Collaboration North East and North Cumbria (ARC NENC – NIHR200173); LM and SK are funded by the NIHR Applied Research Collaborations Greater Manchester (ARC GM – NIHR200174); CB is additionally funded by The Wellcome Trust (221266/Z/20/Z), The Health Foundation (2211473) and the NIHR School of Public Health Research (NIHR204000). The views expressed in this publication are those of the author(s) and not necessarily those of The Wellcome Trust, The Health Foundation, National Institute for Health Research, the Department of Health and Social Care, or the Northern Health Science Alliance. We especially thank ARC NENC and ARC GM who funded the open access publication.

Foreword

It was 23 March 2020 when everything finally fell silent. The mist of confusion and panic over what to do about the arrival, and rapid spread, of a new virus settled and everything finally came to a full stop.

Too late. While the streets were quiet, the virus had spread far and wide. And essential workers went on: supermarket workers, social care workers, petrol station attendants, nurses, and doctors kept on working while COVID-19, already embedded deep in the capital, continued its spread across the UK.

As the pandemic progressed rapidly, then in waves, what public health experts feared and expected happened. COVID-19 spread into those parts of the country which were already suffering from some of the worst inequalities in the Western world.

The North of England has poor health on a huge scale. Its life expectancy ahead of the pandemic was two years less on average than that in the rest of England, and its people spent many more years in ill health. So when COVID-19 hit communities in the North, it quickly became clear that its effects would be devastating and entrenched in the region.

As mortality rates appeared and those grim numbers regularly read out by Professors Whitty and Van Tam became a weekly feature of life, conversations between Professor Bambra, Dr Munford and ourselves came quickly. The previous work we'd done on the 2018 Health for Wealth report had shown the huge health and economic costs of health inequalities in the North. We wondered what the regional impact of COVID-19 would be. The parallels with previous inequalities were striking and delivered a clear story of a 'syndemic' – combining chronic deprivation, long-term ill-health and the novel virus.

Work was produced quickly in the hope that quick analysis of the situation could inform policymakers of the right actions to take. Our rapid analysis in July 2020 was followed by two reports detailing the impact of COVID-19 in the North, then the Child of the North report looking at the situation for children and the parallel pandemic report looking at the impact of COVID-19 on the region's mental health.

There were some successes because of these reports – the link between health inequalities and worse outcomes from COVID-19 drove vaccinators into the North of England for example and questions were asked in both the House of Commons and the House of Lords around the impact of health inequalities and the pandemic. Manchester Metro Mayor Andy Burnham cited our findings in his influential press conferences to illustrate the problems faced in the North.

Fast forward to autumn 2022. The virus is still with us but daily life is much as it was in early 2020 before COVID-19 hit. But we are, particularly in the North of England, now sicker and poorer than pre-pandemic.

The work of the authors of this book shows what happens when a pandemic hits an already sick population. It is an essential record of a moment in time with lessons on population health that should continue to inform policymakers as they examine this period. Pandemics are sadly not new, and most scientists believe that in a hyper-connected and rapidly warming world we are likely to see them more frequently.

This is why this book is so important. We're in a period where we need to take stock and regain the health of the UK population, rebuild our economy and develop resilience to future health shocks.

Understanding where the North of England fits into the rejuvenation of the country is vital. The economic arguments for improving the health of the most deprived communities in the UK is clearly and dramatically shown. The North's relatively poor physical and mental health meant it suffered under the pandemic for longer and it hit harder. Nowhere has it been illustrated more clearly that health is wealth – and that is a lesson we must take into the future.

Hannah Davies and Séamus O'Neill
Northern Health Science Alliance

ONE

North and South: introduction

There is a longstanding and well-established regional health divide in England: on average, people in the Northern region of England live two years less than those in the rest of the country. These geographical divides were exacerbated by austerity and feelings of being 'left behind' are considered to have contributed to the 2016 Brexit vote and spurred the Conservative Party to propose a regional development policy of levelling up as a centre piece of their successful 2019 election manifesto. In 2020, the COVID-19 pandemic hit against this backdrop of severe regional inequality. While the pandemic affected all aspects of life, all people, and all parts of the country, it did not do so equally: the North was hardest hit. This book addresses this vital contemporary issue of regional inequalities through the prism of the impact of the COVID-19 pandemic.

We demonstrate that COVID-19's regional impact has been unequal across three domains: mortality, mental health, and the economy. We also further explore regional inequalities in relation to sex, ethnicity, and income/deprivation. Using original data analysis of a wide range of sources (including health and social care survey data, administrative health care data, mortality data, economic data), we show how the pandemic disproportionately impacted on the three Northern regions of England (North East, North West, and Yorkshire and The Humber), exacerbating existing regional inequalities in health and wealth. It demonstrates that: COVID-19 deaths were higher in the North of England, the North experienced six weeks more in lockdown, higher wage reductions, more furlough, higher unemployment, and worse mental health. We calculate that the unequal regional impact of the pandemic will cost the UK economy over £7 billion in lost productivity due to higher mortality and £2 billion in increased mental ill health.

We will draw on a wide range of interdisciplinary concepts to contextualise our original data analysis. Our book therefore also aims to make a conceptual as well as an empirical contribution to the COVID-19, health inequalities, health geography, and regional economics literatures. We argue that the COVID-19 pandemic interacted with – and exacerbated – longstanding regional inequalities in health and wealth. We conclude by setting out what we can do post-pandemic to reduce inequalities in health and wealth in the future.

This introductory chapter sets out the context of regional inequalities in health and wealth in England before the pandemic. It will provide a brief historical overview of the North; the North–South regional health divide; and regional economic inequalities – as well as exploring the relationships between health and wealth. It will also introduce some of the key conceptual material that underpins the rest of the book including the focus on the North as a distinct region, explanations for geographical inequalities in health (including intersectionality and the amplification of deprivation thesis) and the syndemic pandemic.

The North

First, it is important to define the North of England as this is a key focus of our book.[1] The North–South divide occupies a particular place within the English imagination and the term itself dates back to the 1920s (Russell, 2004).

It first came to prominence in the 19th century as the process of industrialisation started in the North of England. The North therefore typified the problems (and benefits) of industrialisation while the South became associated with rurality and the 'rural idyll'.[2] However, defining the North today is not an uncontroversial task as there are longstanding (and sometimes heated) debates both in academia and among the wider public about where the North is: it has variously been conceptualised as the kingdom of Northumbria, the Humber-Mersey line, the Wash-Severn line, the historical Seven County North (comprising Cheshire, Cumberland, Durham, Lancashire, Northumberland, Westmorland and Yorkshire), the Lowry line or the Administrative North (Bambra, 2016) (Figure 1.1). When reporting data, government agencies divide England into nine regions (North East, North West, Yorkshire and The Humber, South East, the East and West Midlands, the East of England, the South West, and London). The three most northerly of these (North East, North West, Yorkshire, and The Humber) form the so-called Administrative North. We use this three-region definition of the North – partly from a practical perspective (in terms of government data) but also because the Administrative North broadly matches the more colloquial definitions of the North – the Anglo-Saxon kingdom of Northumbria, the Humber-Mersey line and the Seven-County North (Russell, 2004). While not a distinct geopolitical unit today (unlike Scotland or Wales), arguably, there is a longstanding cultural, economic, social – and political – Northern identity (Russell, 2004). The 'North-South divide' has a strong cultural salience today in England – often featuring in popular narratives and discussions. This is because it is part of the longstanding and widely held perception of the North and the South of England as two different countries, two different types of England – divided economically, socially, environmentally, and culturally (Russell, 2004; Dorling, 2011). The North has also developed a distinct identity reflecting the divergent material experience and

Figure 1.1: Dividing lines between North and South

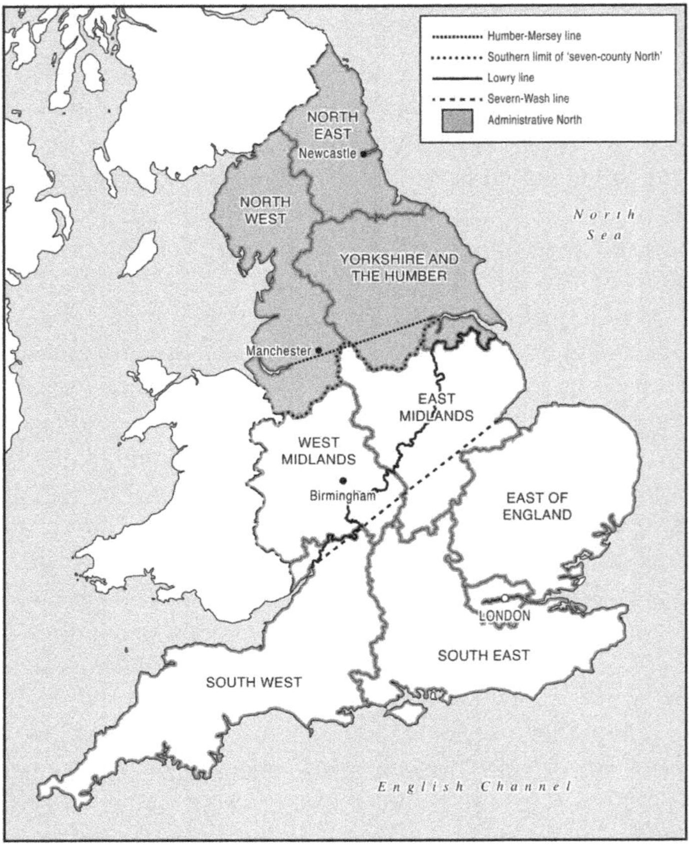

Source: Reproduced under Commons Creative Licence from Bambra (2016)

history of the region and its cultural and political representation (Baker and Billinge, 2004). In recent years, there has been a renewed interest in 'the North' – evident in popular culture, public policy discourse, regional devolution, and political projects such as the Northern Powerhouse initiative, the UK government's post-2019 levelling up strategy, and the establishment of a new 'minister for the North'.

So, taking the Northern regions of England as the North East, the North West and Yorkshire and The Humber, what are they like today? The North East (NE) has suffered from sustained economic decline as industries such as coal mining and ship building have virtually disappeared. There has been very little in the way of new economic activities to replace these old, high employment industries. It has the highest proportion of workless households and deprivation in any English region (Bambra, 2016). The North West (NW) regional economy went through a major period of restructuring and underperformance during the 1980s and 1990s but since then has grown faster than the England average. The region's employment rate though is lower than every other English region except the North East (Bambra, 2016). Yorkshire and The Humber (YH) has also experienced significant economic change, in the 1980s and 1990s the region suffered from decline in its traditional industries in coal mining, steel, engineering, and textiles. However, the region has done relatively well economically, at least in comparison to the NE and NW, in recent years (Bambra, 2016). The three Northern regions have suffered from long-term economic and social decline and as a result have higher rates of deprivation than the rest of England.

Health and wealth in the three Northern regions are discussed further in the following sections.

The North–South health divide

There are deep-rooted and persistent regional inequalities in health across England, with people in the North consistently found to be less healthy than those in the South – across all social groups and among both men and women (Dorling, 2010). Today, there is a two-year life expectancy gap between the North and the rest of England (Table 1.1), and premature death rates are 20 per cent higher for those living in the North across all age groups (Hacking et al, 2011). The North has a significantly higher burden of chronic

Table 1.1: Key health outcomes by English region in 2018/19

	Population (Millions)	Life expectancy at birth (years)		CVD deaths (<75 years /100,000)	Cancer deaths (<75 years /100,000)	Diabetes % (> 17 years)	Obese or overweight % (> =18 years)
		Men	Women				
North	15.5	78.3	82.0	83.8	146.5	7.3	65.1
North East	2.7	77.9	81.7	82.8	152.6	7.4	64.9
North West	7.3	78.3	81.8	86.6	145.6	7.2	64.9
Yorkshire and The Humber	5.5	78.7	82.4	82.0	141.2	7.2	65.4
South	40.5	80.0	83.5	67.8	127.9	6.9	61.8
East Midlands	4.8	79.4	82.9	73.5	133.4	7.3	64.2
West Midlands	5.9	78.9	82.7	78.4	138.4	7.8	65.4
East of England	6.2	80.3	83.7	63.4	126.0	6.9	63.3
South West	5.6	80.2	83.8	61.9	125.6	6.6	61.3

Table 1.1: Key health outcomes by English region in 2018/19 (continued)

	Population (Millions)	Life expectancy at birth (years)		CVD deaths (<75 years /100,000)	Cancer deaths (<75 years /100,000)	Diabetes % (> 17 years)	Obese or overweight % (> =18 years)
London	8.9	80.7	84.5	70.5	120.1	6.6	55.9
South East	9.1	80.7	84.1	59.0	123.6	6.2	60.9
England	56	79.6	83.2	71.7	132.3	6.9	62.3

Source: Public Health England (2020a)

conditions – including: hypertension, diabetes, asthma, chronic obstructive pulmonary disease (COPD), heart, liver and renal disease, cancer, and cardiovascular disease (Table 1.1). There are also higher rates of obesity, alcohol use, and smoking in the North. This 'Northern' health disadvantage has meant that over the last 50 years, 1.5 million Northerners have died earlier than those living in the rest of England (Hacking et al, 2011). Today, England has the highest regional health inequalities in Europe (Bambra et al, 2014a).

By way of example, Figures 1.2 and 1.3 present average life expectancy at birth for both men and women for the stops along some of the major train lines in England: the West Coast Mainline (WCM, a route of 300 miles from London Euston to Carlisle in the North West), the East Coast Mainline (ECM, a route of 335 miles from London Kings Cross to Berwick in the North East), and the Great Western Mainline (GWM, a route of 300 miles from London Paddington to Penzance in the South West) (Bambra and Orton, 2016). The data are geo-referenced to each of the main stations along the routes using the relevant local authority (for example the data for Newark is for Nottinghamshire). The circles represent values above (dark), around (medium), or below (light) the English average of 79.6 years for men and 83.2 years for women.

The visualisations show very clearly the health divides within England, particularly between the North East and South East regions, which have the lowest and highest life expectancies respectively for both men and women. There are gaps of four years for men and five years for women between the best Southern and worst Northern areas. They also demonstrate a socio-spatial gradient, with average life expectancy at birth decreasing the further north the journey takes. There are exceptions to this, with some areas that, while 'Northern' (for example Cheshire), have above average health outcomes.

This health divide has been widening in recent years. Between 1965 and 1995, there was no health gap between younger Northerners aged 20–34 years and their counterparts

Figure 1.2: An English journey: life expectancy for women along the East Coast, Great Western, and West Coast Mainlines

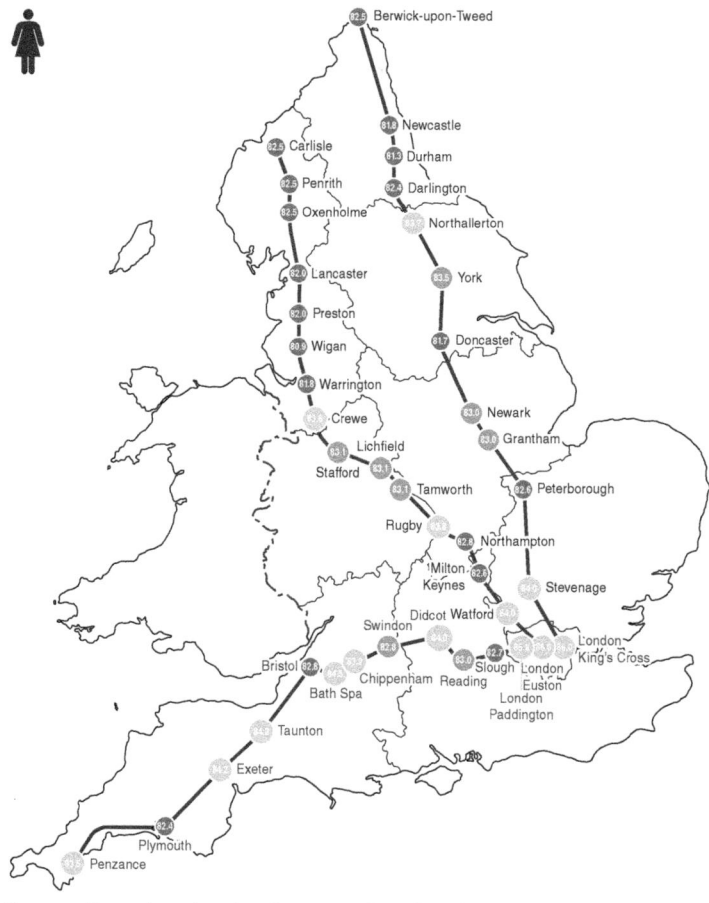

Source: Reproduced under Commons Creative Licence from Bambra and Orton (2016)

in the rest of England. However, mortality is now 20 per cent higher among young people living in the North. Similarly, since 1995, for those aged 35–44 years, excess mortality in the North increased even more sharply to 49 per cent (Buchan et al, 2017). Further, the most deprived local authorities in

Figure 1.3: An English journey: life expectancy for men along the East Coast, Great Western, and West Coast Mainlines

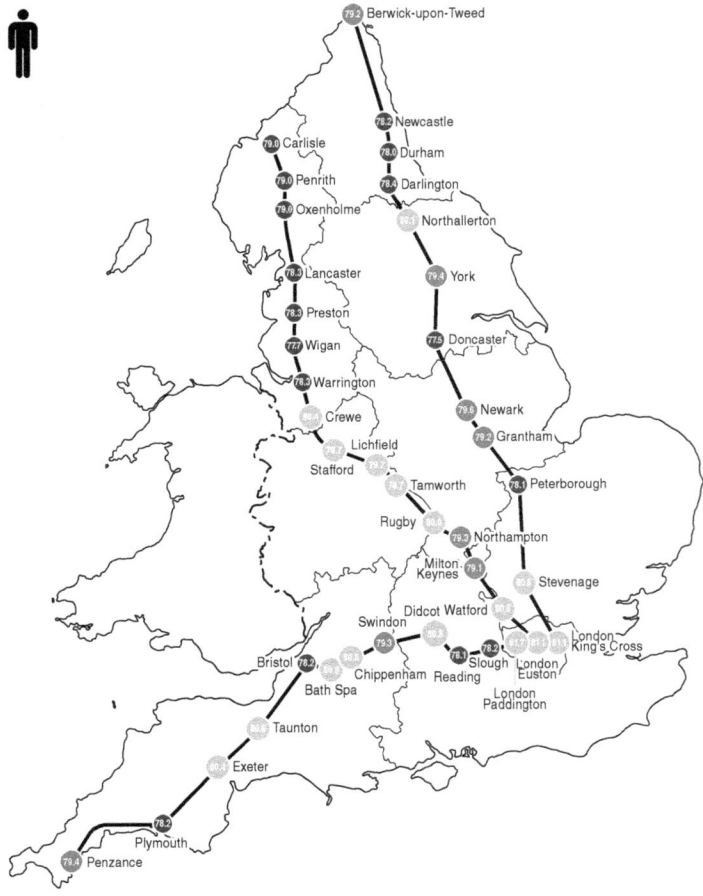

Source: Reproduced under Commons Creative Licence from Bambra and Orton (2016)

the North now have worse health than the most deprived local authorities the rest of England (Whitehead et al, 2014). Figure 1.4 shows how, since 2001, life expectancy in deprived Northern local authorities has improved more slowly than in similar local authorities in the rest of England: on average,

Figure 1.4: Comparison of growth in life expectancy in deprived local authorities in the North and the rest of England since 2001

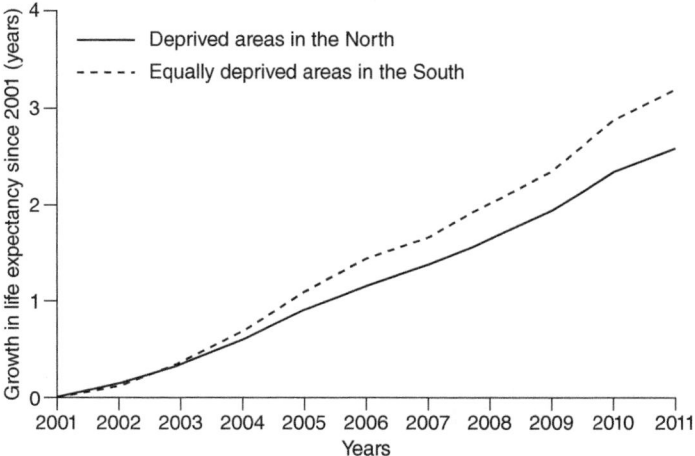

Source: Reproduced under creative commons licence from Whitehead et al (2014)

people living in the most deprived local authorities in the North have a life expectancy of around six months shorter than those in the rest of England. Importantly therefore, even before the pandemic hit, parts of the North had already been falling (even) further behind.

Understanding health and place

Researchers within the field of health geography seek to explain place-based health inequalities like the North–South divide in terms of the interrelation of compositional, contextual, and political economy factors (as visualised in Figure 1.5). This section outlines these theories of 'placing health inequalities'.

The compositional view argues that *who lives here* – primarily the health behaviours (smoking, alcohol, physical activity, diet, drugs), age, ethnic, and socio-economic (income, education, occupation) characteristics of the people living

Figure 1.5: The compass model of health and place

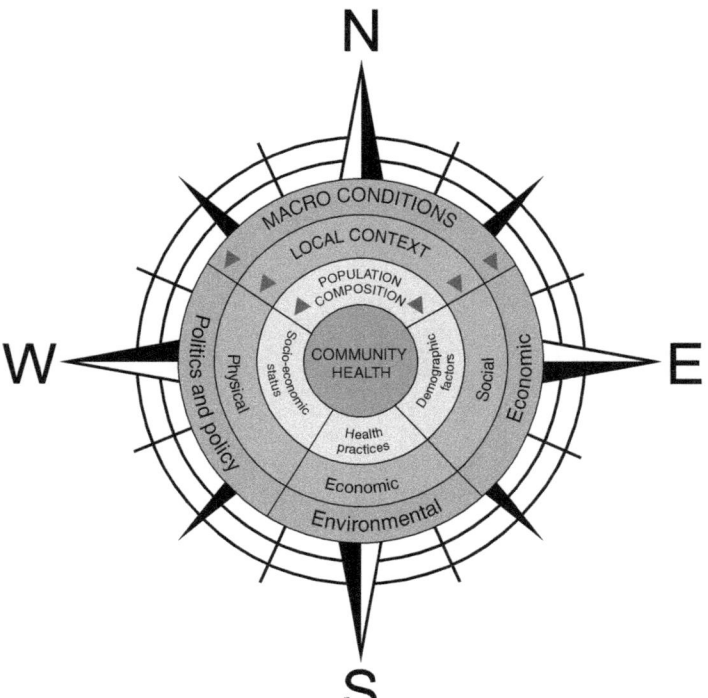

within a particular area (for example a region) determines its health outcomes (innermost 'population composition' ring, Figure 1.5).

It is well established that risky health behaviours such as smoking, alcohol consumption, low physical activity, poor diet, and drug use, all influence health significantly. For example, smoking is the most important preventable cause of mortality in the UK and is causally linked to most major diseases such as cancer and cardiovascular disease (WHO, 2022). So, on average, regions with higher rates of these unhealthy behaviours among their populations would have worse health than others, all things being equal.

The socio-economic status (SES) of people living in an area is also of huge health significance.[3] People with higher occupational status, income or education have better health outcomes, higher life expectancy and lower mortality rates than those from lower SES backgrounds. This is because people from lower SES backgrounds are less likely to live in good quality housing, have time and money for leisure activities, feel secure at home or work, have good quality work or a job at all, or afford to eat healthy food (Marmot, 2020). These social determinants of health impact on health inequalities through three main *pathways*: materialist, psychosocial, and behavioural/cultural (Bartley, 2016; Skalická et al, 2009).[4] On average, places with more residents from lower socio-economic backgrounds will have worse health outcomes.

The contextual approach alternatively highlights the fact that what *a place is like* also matters for the health of that place ('local context' ring, Figure 1.5). Place mediates the way in which individuals experience the social, economic, and physical processes on their health: places can be salutogenic (health promoting) or pathogenic (health damaging) environments. There are four contextual aspects to place that have traditionally been considered as important to health: economic, social, cultural, and physical:

- Area-economic factors that influence health are often summarised as economic deprivation. They include area poverty rates, unemployment rates, wages, and types of work and employment in the area. The mechanisms whereby the economic profile of a local area impacts on health are multiple. For example, it affects the nature of work that an individual can access in that place (regardless of their own socio-economic position). It also impacts on the services available in a local area, as more affluent areas will attract different services (such as food available locally or physical activity opportunities) than more deprived areas. Area-level economic factors such as poverty are a key predictor of health including cardiovascular disease, all-cause mortality, limiting long-term illness, and health-related behaviours (Macintyre, 2007).

- Places also have social aspects which impact on health. Opportunity structures are the socially constructed and patterned features of the area which may promote health through the possibilities they provide (Macintyre et al, 2002). These include the services provided, publicly or privately, to support people in their daily lives such as childcare, transport, food availability, or access to a family physician or hospital, as well as the availability of health promoting environments at home (for example good housing quality, access and affordability), work (good quality work), and education (such as high quality schools). For example, local environments can shape our access to healthy – and unhealthy – goods and services thus enhancing or reducing our opportunities to engage in healthy or unhealthy behaviours (Pearce et al, 2007).

- There are various cultural aspects of place that impact on health. These include collective social functioning and practices such as levels of social cohesion and social capital within the community (Hawe and Shiell, 2000). Some studies have found that areas with higher levels of social capital have better health such as lower mortality rates, self-rated health, mental health, and health behaviours. More negative collective effects can also come from the reputation of an area (for example, stigmatised places can result in feelings of alienation and worthlessness) or the history of an area (for example, if there has been a history of racial oppression) (Halliday et al, 2021). Place attachment (an emotional bond that individuals or groups have with specific places) in contrast can have a protective health effect (Gatrell and Elliot, 2009). Local attitudes, say around smoking, can also influence health and health behaviours either negatively or positively (Thompson et al, 2007).

- The physical environment is also an important contextual determinant of health and health inequalities. Access to green space (such as parks) can have positive health effects, while negative health effects have been associated with waste facilities, brownfield, or contaminated land as well as air pollution (Bambra, 2016). For example, it has been estimated that air pollution levels in London account for up to 10,000 unnecessary deaths per year (Walton et al, 2015). Similarly, neighbourhoods with larger amounts of brownfield land have higher rates of poor health and limiting long term illness (Bambra et al, 2014b).

Much of the so-called 'neighbourhood effects' literature in social epidemiology has been concerned with distinguishing between contextual and compositional effects (Cummins et al, 2007). Authors often grapple with trying to demonstrate whether the health of the population of a particular place is poor because of the qualities of that place, or whether people with poor health have moved to that place due to lower housing costs for example.

However, the contextual and compositional explanations for how place relates to health are not mutually exclusive (Macintyre et al, 2002): the characteristics of individuals are influenced by the characteristics of the area. They interact – relationally (arrows, Figure 1.5) (Cummins et al, 2007). For example, occupational class can be affected by local school quality and the availability of jobs in the local labour market or children might not play outside due to not having a private garden (a *compositional* resource), because there are no public parks or transport to get to them (a *contextual* resource) or because it might not be seen as appropriate for them to do so (*contextual* social functioning) (Macintyre et al, 2002). Similarly, areas with more successful economies (for example more high-paid jobs) will have lower proportions of lower socio-economic status residents. Further, the collective resources model suggests that all residents, and particularly those on a low income, enjoy better health when they live in areas characterised by more/better social and economic collective resources. This may be especially important for those on low incomes as they are usually more reliant on local services. Conversely, the health of poorer people may suffer even more if they live in a deprived area where collective resources and social structures are limited, a concept known as deprivation amplification: that the health effects of individual deprivation, such as lower SES, can therefore be *amplified* by area deprivation (Macintyre, 2007). So, the deprivation amplification hypothesis asserts that the negative health effects of individual-level low SES (composition) are amplified (relational) for those living in more deprived areas (context) (Macintyre et al, 1993). For example, some studies have found that individual SES inequalities in physical activity are higher in more deprived areas (Macintyre et al, 2008).

The political economy approach to explaining health and place looks beyond the individual and the local environment and focuses instead on the social, political, and economic structures and relations that may be, and often are, outside the control of the individuals or the local areas they affect (outermost, 'macro conditions' ring, Figure 1.5) (Bambra et al, 2019). Individual and collective social and economic factors such as housing, income, and employment – indeed many of the issues that dominate political life – are key determinants of health and wellbeing (Bambra et al, 2005). Why some places and people are consistently privileged while others are consistently marginalised is a political choice – it is about where the power lies and in whose interests that power is exercised. Political choices can thereby be seen as the *causes of the causes of the causes* of geographical inequalities in health (Bambra, 2016). In this sense, geographical patterns of health and disease are produced by the structures, values, and priorities of political and economic systems (Krieger, 2003). Area-level health is determined, at least in part, by the wider political, social, and economic system and the actions of the state (government) and international level actors (supra-national government bodies such as the European Union, inter-state trade agreements as well as the actions of large corporations): politics can make us sick – or healthy (Schrecker and Bambra, 2015). Politics and the balance of power between key political groups – notably labour and capital – determine the role of the state and other agencies in relation to health and whether there are collective interventions to improve health and reduce health inequalities, and also whether these interventions are individually, environmentally, or structurally focused. In this way, politics (broadly understood) is the fundamental determinant of health divides because it shapes the wider social, economic, and physical environment and the social and spatial distribution of salutogenic and pathogenic factors both collectively and individually (Bambra, 2016).

The final theory we draw upon in this book is that of *intersectionality*. Intersectionality was coined by Kimberlé Crenshaw and was further developed by Black feminist researchers and activists as a way to conceptualise the multiple disadvantage experienced by Black women (Crenshaw, 1989, 1991; Collins, 2002; Davis, 1983; hooks, 1981). It is concerned with how interlocking systems of power and structural inequalities serve to oppress those at multiply marginalised intersections of social identities. Intersectionality considers that social categories (for example SES, gender, race, or sexuality) are mutually constructed and together lead to complex experiences of social inequalities. Inequalities vary historically, are culturally specific and vary across time and space (Gkiouleka et al, 2018). People are differentially located within a matrix of power, privilege and disadvantage (Yuval-Davis, 2015) – there is not a single, static social hierarchy in which one aspect of social position (for example social deprivation) is more important than another (Crenshaw, 1992). Different social categories (for example race, gender) interlink in shaping individual experiences – and health outcomes. Social groups, therefore, experience different amounts of disadvantage and privilege associated with their different characteristics – and related to their specific context (Nash, 2008). Groups might experience the benefits of privilege related to one system of power and stratification (for example advantage of whiteness in terms of race/ethnicity), while simultaneously engendering disadvantage of another (for example women in terms of gender roles) (Iyer et al, 2008; Nash, 2008).

Intersectionality has influenced scholarship in various fields including social geography (for an overview see Hopkins, 2019). More recently, a quantitative approach to the study of intersectionality has begun to be adopted by a range of other disciplines, including epidemiology, psychology, and public health (see Bauer et al, 2021). This represents a valuable opportunity to move beyond the 'single-axis' approach commonly taken in these fields (Bauer, 2014), whereby the primary research question is typically centred around just one dimension of social identity, such as gender for example. Following this 'intersectional turn', it has been argued that place should be considered as an aspect of intersectionality (Bambra, 2022) and studies taking this approach are now beginning to emerge (Holman et al, 2022). Employing an intersectional approach in our study of place-based inequalities in the COVID-19 pandemic in specific population groups may help us to better understand why inequalities exist and how we might begin to address them.

This book will draw on these theories of health and place to aid our understanding of our empirical findings on the unequal regional impact of the COVID-19 pandemic.

The regional wealth divide

The previous section outlined how researchers have tried to understand and explain the North–South health divide. A large explanatory factor is the economic divide between the North and the rest of England. This section provides a brief overview of the state of the Northern economy in the decades immediately preceding the pandemic.

While the North–South economic and health divides can be dated back to at least the early 19th century, since the 1980s, they have become much more pronounced with the North faring worse in relative terms than at any point since the Second World War (Bambra, 2016).[5] This increase in regional inequalities has resulted from the dominance of neoliberal economic and social policies implemented by various governments over the last four decades (Schrecker and Bambra, 2015; Bambra, 2016). The post-war Keynesian consensus ended during the economic crisis of the 1970s (when the UK experienced high inflation, high unemployment and low growth).[6] Neoliberalism emerged as the dominant political and economic ideology. Neoliberalism asserts that: (1) markets are the normal, natural, and preferable way of organising human interaction; (2) the primary function of the state is to ensure the efficient functioning of markets; (3) institutions or policies that lead to outcomes different from those that would be expected from a market require justification (Ward and England, 2007).

The Conservative governments of Margaret Thatcher (1979–1990)[7] represented a key turning point. Through the 1980s and 1990s, they rapidly restructured the economy and the welfare state with the pursuit of low inflation replacing full employment as the driver of economic policy. This period was characterised by rapid deindustrialisation;[8] the privatisation and marketisation of key national industries; increasing entitlement restrictions and reductions to the value of social security benefits;[9] vast reductions in the availability of social housing; income and corporate tax cuts; deregulation of the economy with the promotion of labour market flexibility (for example via anti-trade union laws), supply-side economics and a desire to minimise public social expenditure (Harvey, 2005).[10]

To a greater or lesser extent, neoliberalism has continued as the dominant political ideology of successive UK governments over the last four decades (Schrecker and Bambra, 2015). It was significantly turbo-charged after the 2007/8 financial crisis[11] when the Conservative and Liberal Democrat Coalition (2010–2015) and Conservative-majority (2015 to date) governments implemented austerity (reducing budget deficits in economic downturns by decreasing public expenditure and/or increasing taxes) during the 'Great Recession'. This led to further large-scale cuts to central and local government budgets, limits to National Health Service (NHS) budgets as well as steep reductions in welfare services and benefits (Gamble, 2009). The austerity-led welfare reforms took over £19 billion a year out of the economy (or £470 a year for every adult of working age in the country) (Beatty and Fothergill, 2014). The biggest financial losses were experienced by people in receipt of social security benefits (particularly impacting on disabled people and low-income families with children). Local government (including public health and social care) spending fell by nearly 30 per cent in real terms between 2008 and 2015 in England.

As a result, since the 1980s, there has been a substantial increase in economic insecurity, unemployment, income inequality, poverty, and poor health – particularly in the former industrial heartlands of the North of England.[12] While neoliberalism adversely impacted on all areas of high deprivation, the North of England was particularly vulnerable to its health-damaging effects because it had higher rates of industrial and public sector employment (and trade union membership); higher levels of social housing occupation; higher rates of benefit receipt among the population; and more communities with high rates of deprivation. Likewise, despite the claim by the UK Prime Minister David Cameron when implementing austerity that 'we are all in it together', the Northern post-industrial areas were hardest hit – as more than two-thirds of the 50 local authority districts worst affected by the reforms were in the Northern 'old industrial areas' – places like Blackpool, Liverpool, and Middlesbrough (Beatty and Fothergill, 2014).[13] This backdrop arguably shaped the outcome of key political events including the 2016 Brexit vote – when a large proportion of people in the North voted to leave the European Union – as well as the election of a Conservative majority government in 2019 on the promises of 'getting Brexit done' and 'levelling up' the country.[14]

So, immediately prior to the COVID-19 pandemic – as a result of deindustrialisation, neoliberal economics and austerity, a disproportionate number of Northern communities were characterised by high rates of long-term unemployment, poverty, and low-paid, insecure work: economic inactivity rates were 25.8 per cent in the North East compared to 18.8 per cent in the South East; poverty rates were also over five percentage points higher in the North than the rest of England; job growth since 2004 was less than one per cent in the North compared to over 12 per cent in London, the South East, and the South West; gross value added (GVA) per worker in the North was £4 per hour less than in the rest of England; and average annual earnings were more than 10 per cent lower than the rest of England (Bambra et al, 2018). This has fuelled feelings that the North has been 'left behind' in terms of economic development (Goodwin and Heath, 2016).

So, before the pandemic, the North of England had significantly higher rates of deprivation than the rest of the country. This is illustrated in Figure 1.6 which maps the geographical distribution of deprivation across English local authority district (LAD, left-hand panel) and lower super output areas (LSOA, right-hand panel)[15] using quintiles of deprivation from the 2019 Index of Multiple Deprivation (IMD).[16] It shows that the more deprived areas are much more concentrated in the North (as well as in London), particularly in urban areas. In particular, the North has the highest percentage of LADs within the most deprived fifth quintile: 41 per cent of all LADs within the North are in the most deprived 20 per cent nationally, compared to only 5 per cent of LADs in the rest of the country. The region with the greatest percentage of LADs in the most deprived quintile is the North East (50 per cent). The region with the lowest percentage of LADs in the most deprived quintile is the South West (3 per cent).

Figure 1.6: Deprivation by English local authorities and neighbourhoods (lower super output areas), 2019

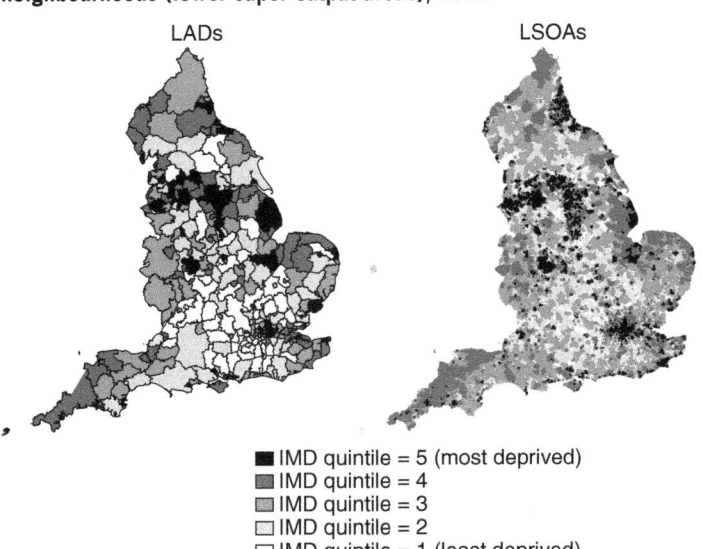

LADs   LSOAs

■ IMD quintile = 5 (most deprived)
▓ IMD quintile = 4
▒ IMD quintile = 3
☐ IMD quintile = 2
☐ IMD quintile = 1 (least deprived)

Conversely, the North has only 6 per cent of its LADs within the least deprived quintile, compared to 31 per cent in the rest of the country. Regionally, the North East has no LADs within the top two quintiles (least deprived 40 per cent) (Munford et al, 2021).

In our 2018 Health for Wealth report, we explored the links between the regional health divide and the regional productivity divide. We found that regional inequalities in health are a key reason for the productivity difference between the North and the rest of England (Bambra et al, 2018). Long-term health conditions lead to economic inactivity, increased risk of job loss, and lower wages. Improving health in the North would lead to substantial economic gains: it would reduce the £4 gap in productivity per-person per-hour between the North and the rest of England by 30 per cent or £1.20 per-person per-hour, generating an additional £13.2 billion in UK gross domestic product (GDP) each year. So, improving health in the North has the strong potential to improve UK productivity.

We explore the unequal regional health and productivity implications of the pandemic in the rest of this book.

Northern exposure

It was against this backdrop of large and increasing regional inequalities in health and wealth that the COVID-19 pandemic hit the UK and the world in 2020. Very quickly, in the very first stages of the pandemic, it became evident – from the experiences of a variety of countries – that there were significant socio-economic and ethnic inequalities in COVID-19 infections, symptom severity, hospitalisation, and deaths (Bambra et al, 2020a; McGowan and Bambra, 2022). In the first wave in England in 2020, for example, deprived areas had death rates more than double those of the most affluent areas (Welsh et al, 2022). Hospitalisation and death rates were also higher among people with certain pre-existing health conditions including hypertension, diabetes, respiratory diseases, heart, liver, renal disease, cancer, cardiovascular disease, obesity, and smoking. The interaction of the pandemic with pre-existing health, social, and economic inequalities has led to COVID-19 being described as a 'syndemic pandemic' (Bambra et al, 2020a; Bambra et al, 2021a). A syndemic exists when risk factors or co-morbidities are intertwined, interactive and cumulative – adversely exacerbating the disease burden and additively increasing its negative effects: 'A syndemic is a set of closely intertwined and mutual enhancing health problems that significantly affect the overall health status of a population within the context of a perpetuating configuration of noxious social conditions' (Singer, 2000: 14).

As the North of England has higher rates of deprivation and a higher burden of chronic disease, we were concerned that COVID-19 would be a regionally unequal pandemic and that the North would be more exposed to its negative health and wealth effects. Working across the NIHR Applied Research Collaborations North East and North Cumbria and Greater Manchester – and supported by our policy partners in the Northern Health Sciences Alliance,[17] we published a series of rapid policy reports empirically examining the impact of the pandemic on the North of England (Bambra et al, 2020b; Munford et al, 2021; Bambra, 2022b; Bambra et al, 2022). This book brings together these analyses – focusing on the unequal regional impact of COVID-19 on mortality, mental health, and the economy. We also place our empirical findings within the wider literature on health and place – arguing that COVID-19 was experienced in the North as a syndemic pandemic; that there is evidence of the amplification of deprivation in the impacts of the pandemic in the North; and that the health inequalities experienced in the North during the pandemic were intersectional.

Chapter Two, The plague year: regional inequalities in deaths from COVID-19: This chapter presents our original analysis of regional differences in COVID-19 mortality in the first year (pre-vaccine) of the pandemic. Using mortality data, we show that COVID-19 deaths were higher in the North of England. We also demonstrate that this higher mortality in the North was not just a case of higher levels of deprivation but a case of deprivation amplification.

Chapter Three, Parallel pandemics: regional inequalities in mental health, hospital pressure, and long COVID: This chapter examines regional trends in the 'parallel pandemics' of mental health, hospital pressure, and long COVID. Using mental health survey data, NHS prescribing data, NHS hospital data, and long COVID prevalence data, we find that these three parallel pandemics have been regionally unequal with worse outcomes in the North. This could cast a long shadow from COVID-19, exacerbating regional health inequalities into the future.

Chapter Four, The costs of COVID-19: regional economic inequalities: This chapter examines the regional impact of the

COVID-19 economic crisis. Through analysing Office for National Statistics (ONS) data we examine regional trends in furlough rates, unemployment rates, and wage levels. We find that the negative economic impacts of the pandemic were higher in the North. We calculate the productivity costs to the UK economy of the higher COVID-19 mortality (Chapter Two), mental health morbidity (Chapter Three), and the harsher lockdown restrictions experienced in the North.

Chapter Five, Perfect storm: understanding the North–South pandemic divide: This discussion chapter places the results from our empirical analyses in Chapters Two to Four within the wider conceptual and empirical context. It sets out how the regional inequalities in health and wealth we have identified during the pandemic reflect longer-term health divides across the country. Drawing on the conceptual material outlined in this introductory chapter, this chapter reflects on why COVID-19 had such an unequal regional impact.

Chapter Six, Levelling up and building back better: conclusion: The book concludes by reflecting on what can be done to reduce health inequalities. Drawing on international case studies of when inequalities in health have been reduced, we outline what public policy response is needed now to reduce regional health inequalities so that they do not increase for future generations and in any future pandemics.

TWO

The plague year: regional inequalities in deaths from COVID-19

Introduction

This chapter presents our original analysis of regional differences in COVID-19 mortality in the first year (pre-vaccine) of the pandemic. In particular, it focuses on differences between the North (North East, North West, and Yorkshire and The Humber) and the rest of England (the other six regions). Using mortality data, we show that COVID-19 deaths were higher in the North of England. We also demonstrate that this higher mortality in the North was not just a result of deprivation. We provide descriptive analysis of differences in mortality rates and then go on to implement linear regression models where we account for factors known to be associated with increased mortality. We first add in known confounders and then potential mediators and examine the attenuation in the 'North' effect to see what percentage of the difference in mortality between the North and rest of England is potentially preventable as it is attributable to modifiable factors, such as deprivation/poverty and worse pre-pandemic health.

We show that the North experienced significantly higher mortality rates, in both COVID-19 and all-cause, than the rest of England across the whole 13 months of the pandemic. On average, the rates of mortality attributable to COVID-19 during the first 13 months of the pandemic (March 2020 to March 2021) were higher in the North than in the rest of the country: 29.4 more people per 100,000 died of COVID-19 in the North (204.1 per 100,000) compared to the rest of England (174.4 per 100,000). This represents a 17 per cent higher mortality rate in the North compared to the rest of England.

These regional inequalities persisted even after we account for the age structure and ethnic composition of the populations, underlying deprivation, and the proportion of high-risk individuals shielding (as a proxy for underlying health status). 51 per cent of the increased COVID-19 mortality in the North (or 15 deaths per 100,000) were explained by higher deprivation and worse pre-pandemic health in the North, which are potentially preventable. Even after accounting for higher prevalence of deprivation and worse underlying health, other regional differences remain, making the North more susceptible to adverse health shocks such as pandemics.

We then go on to further explore the effect of deprivation in the North. We show that the North has more deprived areas and higher COVID-19 mortality rates. We additionally explore the 'deprivation amplification' hypothesis and find evidence that the most deprived areas in the North did worse than equally deprived areas in the rest of England.

Taken as a whole, the results in this chapter paint a worrying picture for the North of England. They highlight the need for the levelling up of regional inequalities to be pushed further up the government's agenda. If levelling up had occurred pre-pandemic, we estimate that around 2,500 Northern deaths due to COVID-19 could, and should, have been prevented.

Methods

We used the COVID-19 age standardised mortality rates (reported per 100,000 population) reported by the ONS.[1]

The data are available for each month from March 2020 to March 2021[2] and for the combined 13 month period. Here we focus on deaths attributable to COVID-19.[3] COVID-19 age standardised mortality rates are available at various geographical levels, from country down to LADs. Here, we use data for regions and for LADs.

We obtained demographic information on the population of each LAD from NOMIS, the ONS's online data portal. We obtained information on the age structure and ethnic structure of each LAD.[4] We did this as there was evidence that COVID-19 was more prevalent in particular ages and ethnicities (Nazroo and Bécares, 2020; Katikireddi et al, 2021). Deprivation was assessed using the 2019 version of the IMD obtained for each LAD from the ONS. IMD is the most commonly used measure of area-level deprivation in England. It produces a ranking of areas in England based on relative local scores for: income, employment, health, education, crime, access to services, and living environment (Department for Communities and Local Government, 2019). To obtain LAD scores and ranks from data available at lower-layer super output area (LSOA) level, population weighted average score of LSOAs within each LAD were calculated. Each LAD was then ranked from one (least deprived) to 308 (most deprived). For ease, we split deprivation into five quintiles ranging from one (least deprived 20 per cent of LADs) to five (most deprived 20 per cent of LADs). We additionally obtained information on the number of people who were 'shielding' per 10,000 in each LAD. In 2020, the UK government advised certain groups of people who were perceived to be more vulnerable to COVID-19 to shield, or further reduce their contacts with other people.[5] These data were available from NHS Digital (NHS Digital, 2021).[6]

The main hypothesis we tested was that mortality rates will be higher in the North, but that this 'northern excess

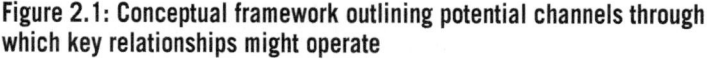

Figure 2.1: Conceptual framework outlining potential channels through which key relationships might operate

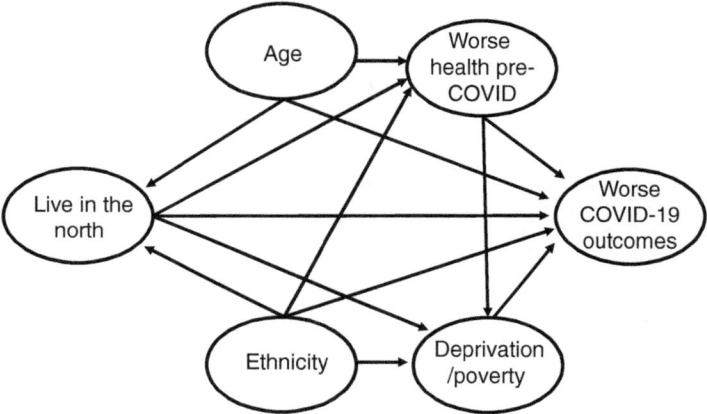

mortality' should become smaller when population and health status (composition – Chapter One) are considered, and smaller still when area-level deprivation (context – Chapter One) is included. To test these hypotheses, we estimated several models informed by a conceptual framework, shown in Figure 2.1.

In the conceptual framework, the key exposure is 'live in the North' and the key outcome is the COVID-19 mortality rates. Age and ethnicity are control variables, known to be associated with both living in the North and worse outcomes. However, deprivation/poverty and worse health pre-COVID-19 are potential mediators – in other words, they could potentially explain the mechanisms by which individuals living in the north may experience worse COVID-19 outcomes.

To obtain estimates for the 'excess' Northern COVID-19 mortality we ran a series of linear regression models and obtained the key parameter estimates.[7] The key parameter in each model is β; it tells us if the mortality rates are statistically different in the North when compared to the rest of England. The later models tell us if this difference persists even after we account for known factors that are associated with mortality rates. We perform all four models with the comparison group between the North and the rest of England. If we assume that the attenuation of the β coefficient for the North on addition of deprivation is indicative of mediation, then this suggests that X per cent of the excess deaths may be explained by the higher levels of deprivation in the North, which are potentially avoidable. That is, to examine the extent to which the higher mortality rates in the North were potentially avoidable, we compare the size of β in Model 3 to Model 4.

Ethnicity may also be thought of as a potential mediator in the relationship between living in the North and experiencing worse COVID-19 outcomes (not shown in Figure 2.1), rather than a confounder, and hence we estimate models where ethnicity can be thought of as either a confounder (Model 3) or as solely a mediator (model 4). We therefore additionally compare the β term in Model 2 to Model 4.

To ease interpretation, we present the results of the statistical models as graphics. In each case, the size of the bar represents the magnitude of the estimated coefficient β. The lines represent the 95 per cent confidence intervals.

Results

COVID-19 mortality rates by region and selected Northern areas

Figure 2.2 shows the COVID-19 mortality rates for each of the nine regions of England as well as the national average (panel a) and the COVID-19 mortality rates for selected Northern Metropolitan Areas and Counties (panel b).

Regionally, during the first 13 months of the pandemic, the North West (233.7 per 100,000) and North East (212.8 per 100,000) had the second and fourth highest COVID-19

Figure 2.2: COVID-19 mortality rates per 100,000 (March 2020 to March 2021)

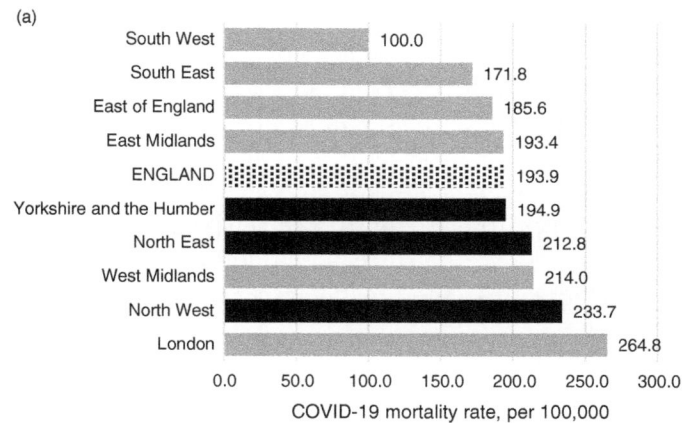

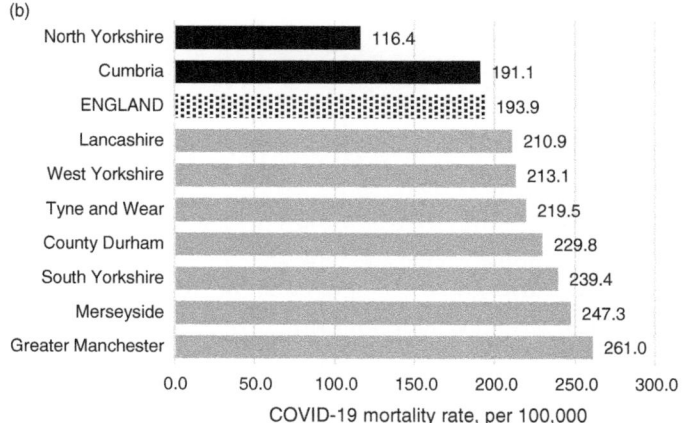

Note: In panel (a), the three regions in the North are coloured black. The remaining nine regions in the rest of England are coloured grey. The English average in shown as a hashed bar. In panel (b), the bars coloured black indicate mortality rates above the English average. The bars coloured grey indicate mortality rates below the English average.

mortality rates, respectively (Figure 2.1, panel [a]). Yorkshire and The Humber had the fifth highest COVID-19 mortality rate (194.9 per 100,000). London had the highest COVID-19 mortality rate (264.8 per 100,000). The South West (100.0 per 100,000) and the South East (171.8 per 100,000) had the lowest and second lowest COVID-19 mortality rates, respectively. Regionally, the COVID-19 mortality rate in the North West was 39.8 per 100,000, or 21 per cent higher than the English average; 18.9 per 100,000, or 10 per cent higher than the English average in the North East; and 1.0 per 100,000, or 1 per cent higher than the English average in Yorkshire and The Humber.

Almost all counties and metropolitan areas in the North had higher mortality than the national average (Figure 2.2, panel [b]). For example, the COVID-19 mortality rate in:

- Greater Manchester was 67.1 per 100,000, or 35 per cent higher than the English average.
- Merseyside was 53.4 per 100,000, or 28 per cent higher than the English average.
- South Yorkshire was 45.5 per 100,000, or 24 per cent higher than the English average.
- County Durham was 35.9 per 100,000, or 19 per cent higher than the English average.
- Tyne and Wear was 25.6 per 100,000, or 13 per cent higher than the English average.
- West Yorkshire was 19.2 per 100,000, or ten per cent higher than the English average.
- Lancashire was 17.0 per 100,000, or nine per cent higher than the English average.

However, in Cumbria (2.8 per 100,000 fewer deaths, or one per cent lower) and North Yorkshire (77.5 per 100,000 fewer deaths, or 40 per cent lower) COVID-19 mortality was lower than the national average.

Excess COVID-19 mortality in the North

The analysis in the previous subsection showed that there was, on average, higher COVID-19 mortality in the North, compared to the rest of England. However, it is not clear from this what percentage of the increased mortality suffered in the North was attributable to factors such as different population structures and prevalence of deprivation. Here, we analyse the relationship between COVID-19 mortality rates and population characteristics, as well as modifiable factors such as deprivation and the underlying health status of the population.

Figure 2.3 presents the results for the COVID-19 mortality rates during the first 13 months of the pandemic.[8] During the pandemic, the COVID-19 mortality rate in the North is always statistically significantly higher than in the rest of England. This is true even after accounting for the full set of variables listed earlier.

Figure 2.3: Additional COVID-19 mortality (March 2020 to March 2021) in the North, per 100,000

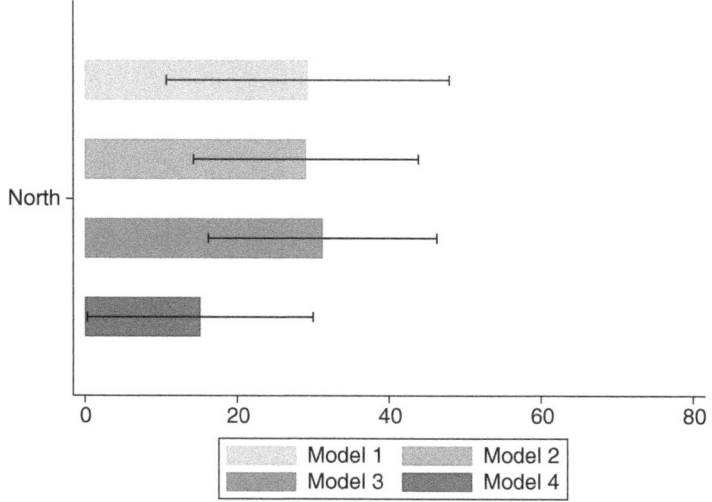

In the unadjusted model (Model 1): 29.4 more people per 100,000 (95% CI: 10.7 to 48.0) died of COVID-19 in the North than in the rest of England (204.1 compared to 174.7 per 100,000, an increase of 17 per cent). When we account for factors known to be associated with higher mortality: in Model 3, where we account for the age and ethnic composition of the populations, 31.3 more people per 100,000 (95% CI: 16.2 to 46.3) died of COVID-19 in the North than in the rest of England; in Model 4, when we added in the mediating variables (deprivation and the proportion of people shielding), 15.2 more people per 100,000 (95% CI: 0.3 to 30.0) died of COVID-19 in the North than in the rest of England. Even after accounting for age, ethnicity, deprivation, and the rate of people shielding, the COVID-19 mortality rate is higher in the North and this difference is statistically significant. The attenuation between Model 1 and Model 4 is 48 per cent.[9] This indicates that 48 per cent of the increased COVID-19 mortality in the North can be explained by observable factors and 52 per cent remains unexplained. When we compare the estimates between Model 3 and Model 4, the attenuation is 51 per cent. Given the conceptual framework reported in Figure 2.1, we infer here that after ethnicity and age have been accounted for, the remaining 51 per cent of increased mortality in the North was potentially preventable. If deprivation and health in the North were at similar levels pre-pandemic to the rest of England, then 51 per cent of the increased northern COVID-19 mortality – or 15 COVID-19 deaths per 100,000 – could have been prevented.

Deprivation and excess COVID-19 mortality in the North

We showed previously that deprivation was an important factor in explaining COVID-19 mortality. However, it could not completely explain the differences in COVID-19 mortality between the North and the rest of England. Here we explore

Figure 2.4: COVID-19 mortality rate (March 2020 to March 2021) and area deprivation for local authority districts in England

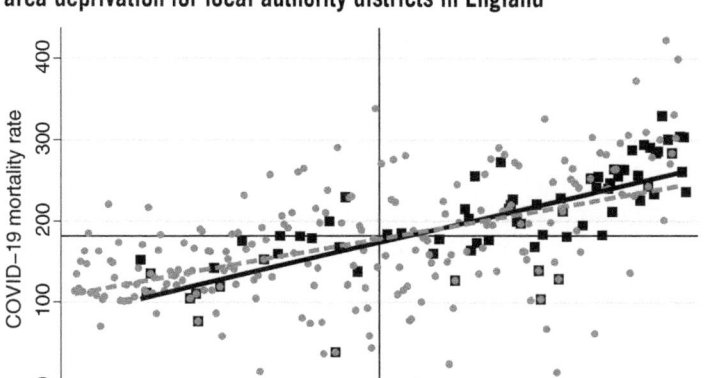

further the different effects that deprivation has in the North and the rest of England.

We present scatter plots of COVID-19 mortality rates against the rank of the LAD by the IMD (higher scores equate to greater deprivation) to analyse the strength of association between mortality rates and deprivation. We show these associations in the North and the rest of England by using different symbols (Figure 2.4). There is a clear positive association between deprivation and mortality, indicating that more deprived areas were likely to suffer higher mortality rates. The gradient of the line of best fit is steeper in the North than it is in the rest of England. The strength of the association between IMD rank and COVID-19 mortality rates is stronger in the North (coefficient=0.58; 95% CI: 0.46 to 0.70) than it is in the rest of England (coefficient=0.44; 95% CI: 0.34 to 0.54). The variation explained by the model is also higher in the North ($R^2 = 0.58$) than it is in the rest of England ($R^2 = 0.27$).

In Figure 2.5, we show the number of LADs in the North and the rest of England in each of the four quadrants (high/low deprivation and high/low mortality).[10] The North East quadrant (most deprivation and high mortality rates) can be thought of as being the 'worst' quadrant to be in, whereas the South West quadrant (least deprivation and low mortality rates) can be thought of as being the 'best' quadrant to be in.

From Figure 2.5 it can be seen that in the North, 58 per cent of LADs are in the worst quadrant (that is, have higher than average deprivation and higher than average COVID-19 mortality) compared to 27 per cent of LADs in the rest of England. Conversely, 42 per cent of LADs in the rest of England are in the best quadrant (that is, have lower than average deprivation and lower than average COVID-19 mortality), compared to 24 per cent of LADs in the North.

Deprivation amplification in the north

As noted in Chapter One, the deprivation amplification hypothesis asserts that the negative health effects of individual-level low SES (composition) are amplified (relational) for those living in more deprived areas (context). In the literature, this concept has largely been applied to examining whether differential access to resources (context) between local areas impacts on the relationship between low SES (compositional) and health. However, deprivation amplification has seldom been used to explore interactions between different scales of place – for example by examining differences in the health profiles of more deprived neighbourhoods or local authorities within more – or less – deprived regions. Here, we investigate deprivation amplification in the context of the COVID-19 pandemic. We set out to test the deprivation amplification hypothesis and examine whether – or not – COVID-19 mortality rates by deprivation differ by region in England.

To do this, we use middle super output area (MSOA) level COVID-19 mortality data from England – stratified by MSOA

Figure 2.5: The relationship between the 13 month COVID-19 mortality rate and deprivation in the North and the rest of England

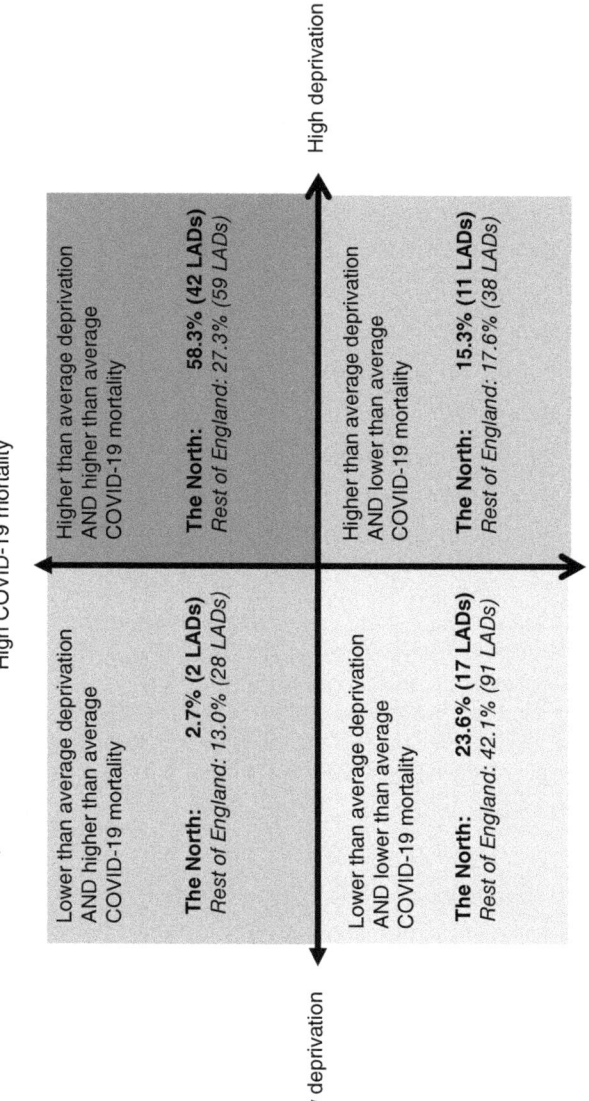

High COVID-19 mortality

Low COVID-19 mortality

High deprivation

Low deprivation

Higher than average deprivation AND higher than average COVID-19 mortality

The North: 58.3% (42 LADs)
Rest of England: 27.3% (59 LADs)

Higher than average deprivation AND lower than average COVID-19 mortality

The North: 15.3% (11 LADs)
Rest of England: 17.6% (38 LADs)

Lower than average deprivation AND higher than average COVID-19 mortality

The North: 2.7% (2 LADs)
Rest of England: 13.0% (28 LADs)

Lower than average deprivation AND lower than average COVID-19 mortality

The North: 23.6% (17 LADs)
Rest of England: 42.1% (91 LADs)

Figure 2.6: Crude COVID-19 mortality rate by IMD quintiles: North vs. the rest of England

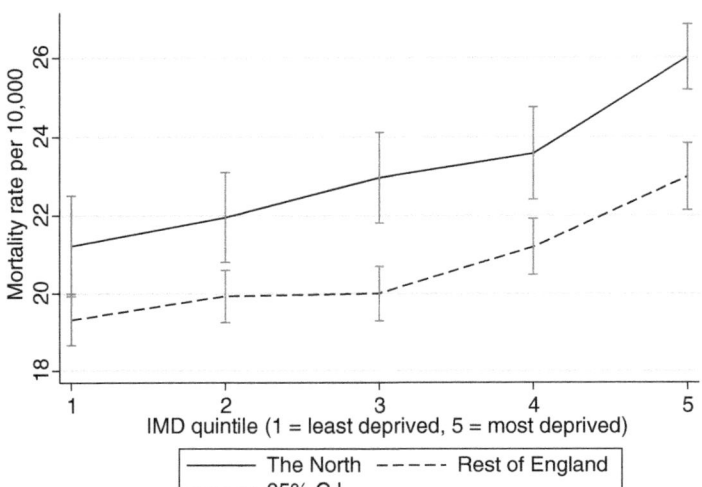

Note: The mortality rate is the population-weighted average of each MSOA within that part of England within that IMD quintile. Each MSOA's mortality rate is defined as the total number of deaths between March 2020 and April 2021 divided by the population estimate from 2019, expressed per 10,000 population. The mortality rates are not age-standardised. In addition, they are 14 month totals, not annual approximations. The 95 per cent confidence interval is calculated by applying the formula mean$\pm 1.96 \times$s.e, where s.e. is the standard error of the mean.

deprivation and by government Office English region.[11] Specifically, it examines whether more deprived MSOAs (the bottom quintile) in more deprived Northern regions suffered greater COVID-19 mortality rates than those in less deprived regions ('the South').

Figure 2.6 shows that MSOAs in the most deprived quintile in the North had higher crude COVID-19 mortality rates than MSOAs in the most deprived quintile in the rest of England, and that this difference was statistically significant (represented by non-overlapping confidence intervals).

Figure 2.7: Conditional COVID-19 mortality rate by IMD quintiles: North vs. the rest of England

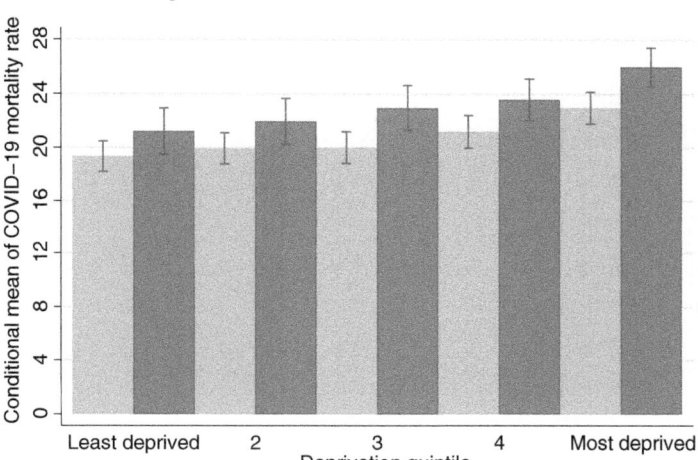

Note: The conditional means are estimated using regression analysis and accounts for the age and ethnicity composition of each MSOA as well as urbanity and deprivation including interactions with the North. The vertical lines are 95 per cent confidence intervals obtained in the traditional way.

This is true for quintiles two, three, and four too. Although MSOAs in the least deprived quintile in the North had higher COVID-19 mortality rates than MSOAs in the least deprived quintile in the rest of England, this difference was not statistically significant.

After accounting for the age and ethnicity structure of MSOAs, deprived MSOAs in the North still had higher average COVID-19 mortality than in the rest of England (Figure 2.7). The most deprived MSOAs in the North had a conditional mean of 26.01 deaths per 10,000 (95% CI: 24.60 to 27.42) compared to 22.98 deaths per 10,000 (95% CI: 21.80 to 24.16) in deprived MSOAs in the rest of England.

We have found that there were regional differences in the effects of deprivation. On average, deprived areas in the North fared worse than equally deprived areas in the rest of England. Our results also show that the higher COVID-19 mortality rates in the North persisted after adjusting for other possible confounding factors (age and ethnicity).

This is the first application of the deprivation amplification concept to the COVID-19 pandemic and our results suggest that there is potentially a deprivation amplification effect regarding geographical inequalities in COVID-19 mortality rates.

Conclusion

This chapter has examined regional COVID-19 mortality rates during the period March 2020 to March 2021 and has shown that, on average, the North fared much worse than the rest of England. COVID-19 mortality rates were statistically significantly higher in the North compared to the rest of England. This remained true even after other factors known to be associated with mortality, such as demographic factors, deprivation, and underlying health status, were accounted for. We estimated that 51 per cent of the increased COVID-19 mortality in the North (or 15 deaths per 100,000) were explained by higher deprivation and worse pre-pandemic health in the North, which are potentially preventable. If regional levelling up had occurred pre-pandemic, and deprivation and health status were equally distributed across the country, we estimate that around 2,500 Northern deaths due to COVID-19 could – and should – have been avoided. Exploring the effects of deprivation further, we show that there is a steeper gradient of the 'deprivation-mortality' curve in the North compared to the rest of England. Far more Northern areas are in the 'highest deprivation – highest COVID-19 mortality rate' quadrant than areas in the rest of England. Finally, we found that the more deprived Northern regions and the more deprived MSOAs across the country had higher COVID-19 mortality rates. We also found that deprived MSOAs in the more deprived Northern regions suffered even greater COVID-19 mortality rates – evidence of the 'deprivation amplification' hypothesis. In the following chapter we go on to examine the wider impacts of the pandemic on mental health, health care and long COVID – the parallel pandemics.

THREE

Parallel pandemics: regional inequalities in mental health, hospital pressure, and long COVID

In this chapter, we examine regional trends in the 'parallel pandemics' of mental health, hospital pressure, and long COVID. For mental health, we use the General Health Questionnaire (GHQ-12) to assess the impact of the pandemic on self-reported mental health in the North. We analyse inequalities in GHQ-12 within the North in terms of sex, ethnicity, income, and age. In addition, we explore the use of mental health services before and during the pandemic by analysing anti-depressant prescribing data – a proxy indicator for the presence of depressive disorders.[1] Finally, we examine regional inequalities in hospital pressure by comparing differences between the North and the rest of England in terms of the proportion of hospital beds occupied by COVID-19 patients, as well as regional variations in the scale of reductions in non–COVID-19 hospital activity during the pandemic.

We show that across the country, mental health declined during the COVID-19 pandemic, with scores at their lowest in January 2021 (approximately a 5 per cent decrease in average GHQ-12 scores across the country compared to 2019). By

September 2021, average mental health scores still had not returned to pre-pandemic levels. This lack of recovery was more pronounced in the Northern regions. Our analyses reveal worse mental health for people from ethnic minority backgrounds and for people aged 15–35 in the North. Further, our analyses by sex, region, and ethnicity show that ethnic minority women living in the North of England had the lowest average mental health scores throughout the pandemic. In addition, our analyses show that the mental health gap between the lowest and highest earners increased four-fold during the pandemic. We then go on to analyse trends in anti-depressant usage. We found that over 20 per cent more anti-depressants were prescribed per person in the North compared to the rest of England in the three years prior to the pandemic. Furthermore, during the pandemic, anti-depressant prescribing increased across the country, but the regional gap also increased.

Finally, in terms of hospital pressures, we show that the North experienced significantly higher bed occupation by COVID-19 patients than the rest of England – and that these regional differences persisted even after accounting for the differing deprivation, age, ethnic, and health conditions of the population. Drawing on data from the Institute of Fiscal Studies (IFS), we also show that, on average, there were greater reductions in non–COVID-19 hospital activity (fewer elective inpatient admissions, fewer non–COVID-19 emergency inpatient admissions, and fewer outpatient appointments) in the North than in the rest of the country during 2020. Using ONS data, we compare regional inequalities in long COVID rates and show that long COVID rates were 30 per cent higher in the North.

Taken as a whole, the results in this chapter suggest that England has experienced several 'parallel pandemics' of poor mental health and increased anti-depressant usage, increased hospital pressure and a greater burden of long COVID. These have adversely impacted the North of England the most and may have long-term consequences for future regional health inequalities.

Regional trends in self-reported mental health

Research into mental health in England during the most intense period of the pandemic and associated periods of lockdown suggests that a decline in mental health was experienced by many, across many parts of the country (Fancourt et al, 2021; Office for National Statistics, 2021; Daly et al, 2020). Further to this, several studies have demonstrated inequalities in mental health during the pandemic – with COVID-19 particularly impacting the mental health of women (O'Connor et al, 2021, Daly et al, 2020), ethnic minorities (Proto and Quintana-Domeque, 2021; Niedzwiedz et al, 2021), and young people (O'Connor et al, 2021; Saunders et al, 2021; Pierce et al, 2020). However, despite the well-established existence of regional inequalities in terms of health outcomes, access to resources and indeed the different region-specific lockdown periods and economic impacts (Chapter Four), little focus has yet been placed on investigating these inequalities by region or the intersectional impact of region-specific inequalities in mental health during the COVID-19 pandemic. In this chapter, we address this gap.

Our first analysis used data from the nationally representative UK Household Longitudinal Survey (UKHLS; also known as *Understanding Society*).[2] This survey has sample of around 100,000 individuals living in around 40,000 households. The survey collects information on a range of topics, including mental and physical health, socio-economic position, and demographic characteristics.[3] Survey data covering the period from January 2019 to December 2019 was used as a pre-COVID-19 baseline and compared to the nine waves of the COVID-19 survey (April 2020–Sept 2021).[4] Participants in the COVID-19 survey were linked to their baseline pre-COVID-19 data from 2019. The sample size for England for each of the COVID-19 survey waves ranged from 9,686 to 14,425 people.

We used the 12-item version of the General Health Questionnaire (GHQ-12) on a scale from zero to 36 to assess non-psychotic mental ill health (such as anxiety and depression) with higher values indicating better mental health.[5] This scale can also be used in a 'caseness' approach – whereby a score greater than or equal to 4 is understood to indicate the probable presence of a diagnosable mental health disorder.[6] In terms of the coding of relevant covariates, age was categorised into three bands: 15–35 years, 36–65 years, and over 66 years. Sex was a binary variable of 'male' or 'female'. Equivalised household income was calculated for both the baseline and COVID-19 data.[7] Educational qualification data was taken from the 2019 baseline survey and qualifications were coded into three categories: GCSE or lower (including no qualifications), A-level, and higher education qualification or above. Due to limitations in sample size, ethnicity was recoded into a binary variable with respondents allocated to White British or ethnic minority categories.[8]

Descriptive statistics were used to present trends over time. The descriptive statistics show that the sample was comprised of a greater proportion of women than men across all regions (55.3 per cent for the overall sample). The largest age category across all regions was 46–55 (range: 16.8 per cent to 20.6 per cent), except in the North East where it was the 56–65 category (20.4 per cent) and the North West where it was the 36–46 group (17.7 per cent). The sample was predominantly White British (74.4 per cent for the overall sample), with the lowest proportion in London (33.0 per cent) and the highest in North East (95.0 per cent). The average annual equivalised household income was £14,812, with the highest average found in London (£17,953) and the lowest in Yorkshire and The Humber (£12,628). Finally, a large proportion of the sample had only a GCSE or lower level education (47.9 per cent). The proportion of people in the lowest category of education was greatest in the North East (56.0 per cent) and lowest in London (36.8 per cent).[9]

Figure 3.1: Trends in GHQ-12 (higher scores indicating better mental health) between 2019 and September 2021 by region

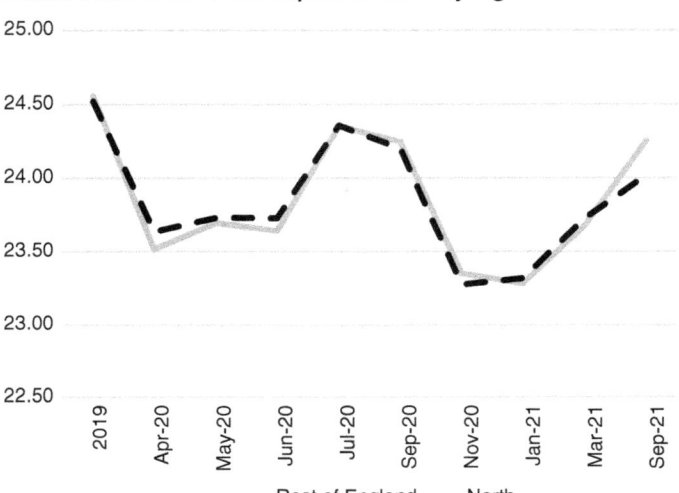

Figure 3.1 shows that before COVID-19 (2019 baseline), all regions had similar GHQ-12 scores (around 24.5). During the pandemic, these scores decreased across all regions during the first year of the pandemic (2020) – indicating worsening mental health: both the North and the rest of England experienced a fall of around 5 per cent in average GHQ-12 mental health scores – with scores at their lowest in January 2021. There were some improvements after January 2021 but even by September 2021, scores had not returned to the pre-pandemic average and were lower by 0.5, or half a point on the GHQ-12 scale (a 2.0 per cent decrease), in the North and 0.3 (a 1.3 per cent decrease) in the rest of England in September 2021 compared to 2019.

In terms of the proportion of people meeting the threshold for a minor mental health disorder ('caseness'), this also increased substantially in 2020 in both the North and the rest of England. In the North it increased from around 19.96 per cent of the sample in 2019 to 28.66 per cent by April 2021, falling back to 20.10 per cent in September 2021. Similarly, in the rest of England it increased from around 19.79 per cent of the population in 2019 to 29.48 per cent by April 2021, falling back to 19.54 per cent in September 2021. There were no significant differences between the North and the rest of England in these trends.

We also compared inequalities in mental health during the pandemic by sex, ethnicity, income, and age for the North compared to the rest of England. On average, women had lower GHQ-12 scores compared to men throughout the COVID-19 pandemic. These trends were similar across the North and the rest of England. The results of a descriptive analysis by ethnicity (White British compared to ethnic minority) are presented in Figure 3.2. This figure shows that, on average, people from ethnic minority backgrounds had similar mental health scores to those from White British backgrounds in 2019. However, average GHQ-12 scores dropped by a larger amount in the ethnic minority group than in the White British group during the pandemic (a fall of 1.6 points on the GHQ-12 scale, compared to 0.9 for the sample as a whole). By region, this fall was greater for those from ethnic minority backgrounds in the North (a fall of 2.3, compared to 1.5 for the rest of England), and these scores remained lower throughout the pandemic. This decrease was particularly pronounced among ethnic minority women (shown in Figure 3.3), with those from the North having the lowest mental health throughout the time series: in the last wave of the COVID-19 survey (September 2021), the average GHQ-12 score for ethnic minority women in the North was 1.6 points lower than the average score of ethnic minority women in the rest of England.

We also assessed inequalities in mental health by income groups in the North, compared to the rest of England. Figure 3.4 shows the trends in mental health, by the top (highest income) and bottom (lowest income) quintiles of equivalised household income. The trends by quintile are

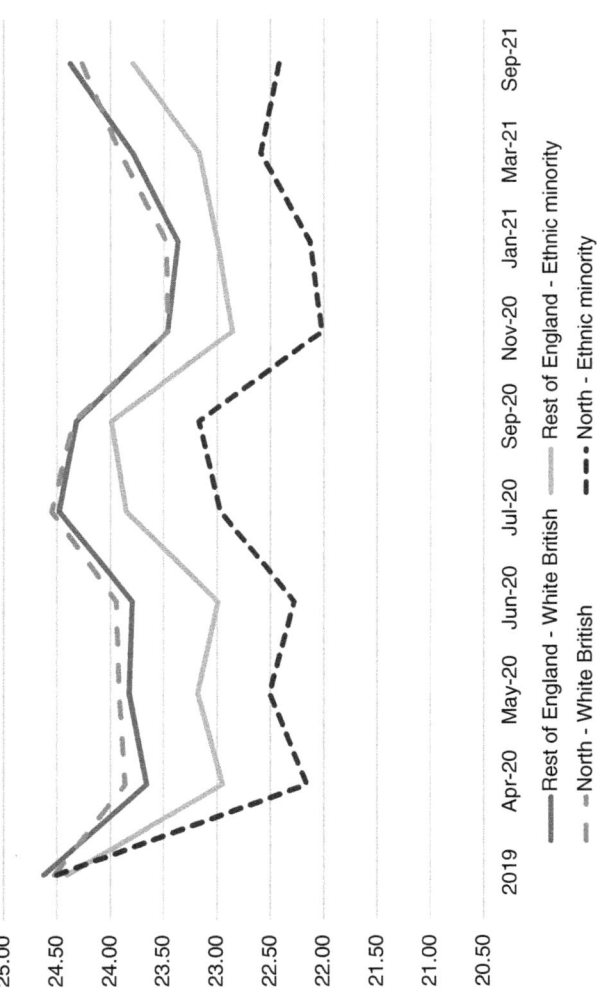

Figure 3.2: Trends in GHQ-12 (higher scores indicating better mental health) between 2019 and September 2021 by region and ethnic group

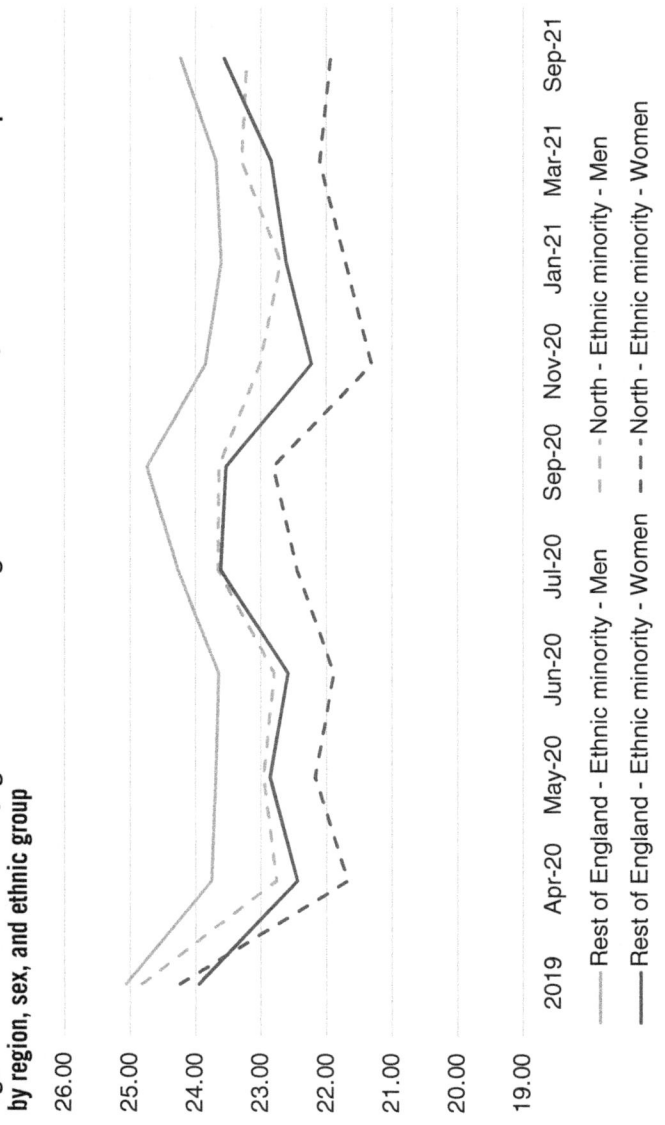

Figure 3.3: Trends in GHQ-12 (higher scores indicating better mental health) between 2019 and September 2021 by region, sex, and ethnic group

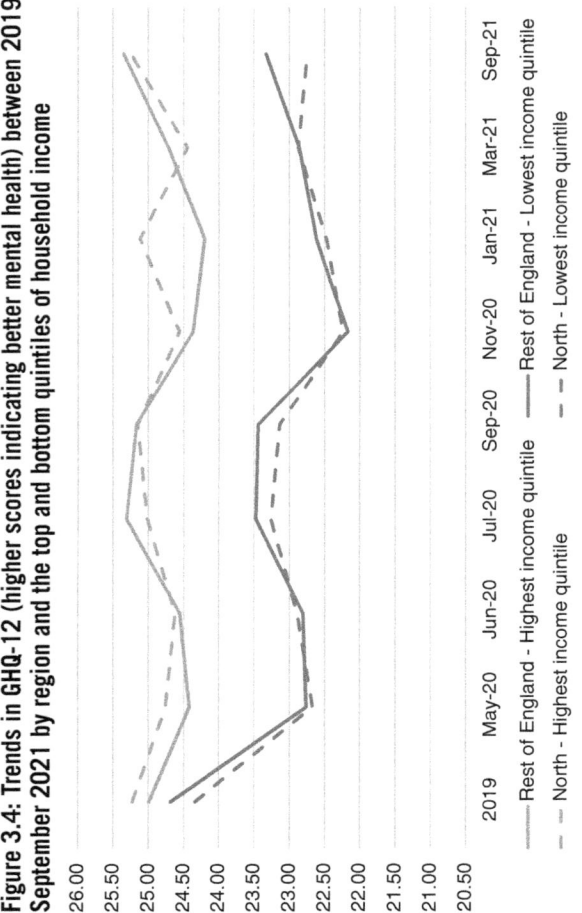

Figure 3.4: Trends in GHQ-12 (higher scores indicating better mental health) between 2019 and September 2021 by region and the top and bottom quintiles of household income

Note: April 2020 is omitted from Figure 3.4. This is due to no household income data being available for the COVID-19 survey participants in the first wave of the survey.

Figure 3.5: Difference in percentage points of those meeting the cut-off for a minor psychiatric disorder by age group, 2019 to September 2021

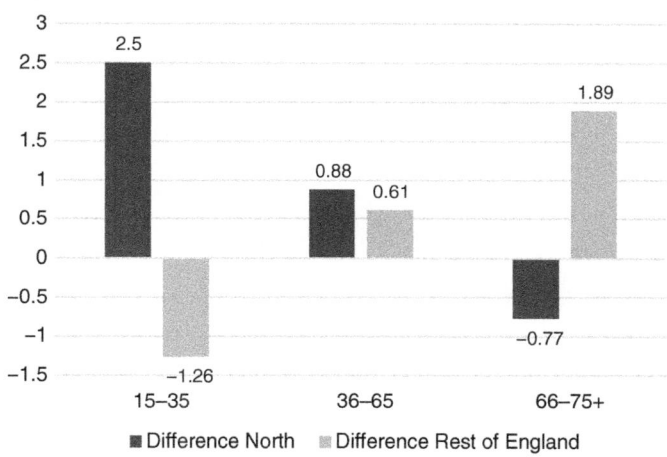

broadly similar in the North and the rest of England. While average mental health scores in the highest income quintile in both parts of the country appeared largely unaffected by the pandemic, average mental health for the lowest income group fell during the pandemic. Importantly, the gap between the lowest and highest quintiles in 2019 was small. However, this gap widened during the pandemic. The mental health gap between the top and bottom income quintiles was larger in September 2021 than it was in 2019 (a difference of 0.47 points on the GHQ-12 scale in 2019, compared to 2.16 points in September 2021 for England overall). This suggests that the pandemic may have widened existing income-based inequalities in mental health.

Figure 3.5 shows the difference in percentage points from 2019 to September 2021 in the proportion of people meeting the cut-off for the potential presence of a minor psychiatric disorder by age group. In both regions, the 36–65 age group had the smallest change between the baseline wave and the final wave of the COVID-19 survey, with an increase of between 0.61 and 0.88 percentage points. The largest increase was in the North for the 15–35 age group (of 2.5 percentage points), whereas this group saw a reduction in the rest of England. The largest increase for the rest of England was the 66–75+ age group (with an increase of 1.89 percentage points), whereas this group saw a reduction in those meeting the threshold in the North.

Regional trends in anti-depressant prescriptions

In our next analysis, we used data coded in the British National Formulary (BNF) directory as an anti-depressant to understand trends in the prescribing of anti-depressants by region.[10] The dataset is a complete record of detailed information relating to prescriptions issued in England. Data are coded at the GP practice level, but are aggregated and released at the Clinical Commissioning Group (CCG) level.[11] The North (consisting of the North West and North East and Yorkshire) contains 51 CCGs whereas the rest of England (consisting of London, Midlands, East of England, South East and South West) contains 55 CCGs.[12] To calculate the rate of anti-depressants prescribed per person we used the total quantity of prescriptions and population sizes in CCGs. Using per-person measures accounts for the unequal sizes of CCGs.

We analysed the trends in anti-depressant prescribing over a five-year period consisting of a pre-pandemic period (January 2017 to February 2021) and a 20 month period during the pandemic (defined as March 2020 to November 2021) by region and North versus the rest of England. To investigate if the pandemic had a differential impact on the prescription of anti-depressants in the North of England compared to the rest of England, we implemented a 'difference-in-difference' model.[13] This design allowed us to examine the differential impact of the parallel pandemic by comparing the change in the prescription of anti-depressants from before the pandemic to during the pandemic (observed in the North of England), to the change in the prescription of anti-depressants from before the pandemic to during the pandemic (observed in the rest of England).[14]

In the three years prior to the pandemic, the Northern regions consistently experienced higher levels of anti-depressant prescribing than regions in the rest of England. The North East, Yorkshire and The Humber and the North West had the highest average number of anti-depressant prescribing per person during this period (Table 3.1). This continued during the pandemic, with the average number of anti-depressants prescribed per person standing at 5.39 (North East, Yorkshire, and The Humber) and 5.27 (North West). London and the South East had the lowest rates with average prescriptions per person of 2.16 (pre) and 2.44 (during) and 3.8 (pre) and 4.27 (during), respectively (Table 3.1). Prior to the pandemic, the North had consistently greater numbers of anti-depressant prescriptions per person (4.73) compared to the rest of England (3.86). Anti-depressant prescriptions per person increased during the pandemic in both the North (5.32) and the rest of England (4.37). The difference-in-difference analysis found that the gap between the North and the rest of England increased during the pandemic: the North experienced an additional increase of 0.1 units of anti-depressant prescription (p<0.05, 95% CI: 0.03 to 0.21) compared to the rest of the country.[15] This additional increment experienced in the North is an increase of around 2 per cent in the North on the pre-pandemic level – over and above the increases experienced in the rest of England.

Regional trends in hospital pressure

We obtained the number of hospital beds occupied by COVID-19 patients in NHS Trusts from the COVID-19 NHS Situation Report for the period of April 2020 to

Figure 3.6: Percentage of beds occupied by COVID-19 patients, April 2020 to March 2021

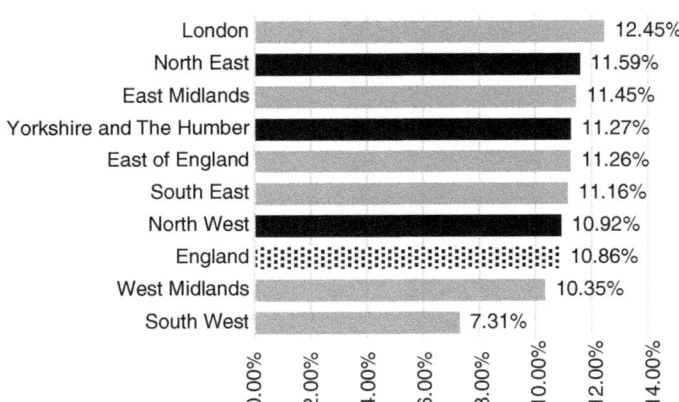

March 2021.[16] The number of beds occupied by COVID-19 patients was calculated as a proportion of the total number of beds. Each NHS Trust was then mapped to a local authority based on the hospital location and then mapped to its region using look-up tables, as well as to the North or the rest of England.

During the first year of the pandemic, the national average for England for beds occupied by COVID-19 patients was 10.9 per cent (Figure 3.6). All three Northern regions were at or above the national average: the North East had 11.6 per cent beds occupied by COVID-19 patients, Yorkshire and The Humber had 11.3 per cent, and the North West had 10.9 per cent. London and had the highest bed occupancy rate at 12.5 per cent, while the South West had the lowest at 7.3 per cent.

However, it is not clear from this descriptive data what percentage of the increased hospital bed occupancy experienced in the North was attributable to differences in population composition (see Chapter One on composition) between the North and the rest of England such as deprivation

Table 3.1: Mean number of anti-depressants prescribed per person between January 2017 and February 2020 (pre-pandemic) and between March 2020 and November 2021 (during the pandemic)

	January 2017 to February 2020 (pre-pandemic)	March 2020 to November 2021 (during the pandemic)
	Mean (std. dev.) (95% conf. interval)	Mean (std. dev.) (95% conf. interval)
North	4.728 (0.273) [4.639 to 4.816]	5.323 (0.221) [5.223 to 5.424]
Rest of England	3.863 (0.222) [3.791 to 3.935]	4.369 (0.178) [4.288 to 4.450]
East of England	4.040 (0.230) [3.965 to 4.114]	4.559 (0.171) [4.4810 to 4.636]
London	2.163 (0.119) [2.124 to 2.202]	2.444 (0.113) [2.393 to 2.496]
Midlands	4.016 (0.245) [3.937 to 4.096]	4.570 (0.196) [4.481 to 4.659]
North East and Yorkshire	4.756 (0.285) [4.664 to 4.849]	5.387 (0.225) [5.285 to 5.489]
North West	4.702 (0.263) [4.617 to 4.787]	5.267 (0.219) [5.167 to 5.366]
South East	3.805 (0.209) [3.737 to 3.873]	4.270 (0.177) [4.190 to 4.351]
South West	4.418 (0.248) [4.337 to 4.498]	5.002 (0.204) [4.909 to 5.095]

age, ethnicity, and underlying health conditions. Therefore, we analysed the relationship between hospital bed occupancy rates and population characteristics to test whether the 'excess' bed occupancy rates in the North become smaller when population characteristics are included. To test this hypothesis, we estimated four statistical models: Model 1 (base), Model 2 (with base and age), Model 3 (base, age and ethnicity), Model 4 (base, age, ethnicity, deprivation, health conditions).[17] We calculated all four models with a comparison between the North and the rest of England.[18]

Our final model (4) shows that during the pandemic period analysed, the percentage of hospital beds occupied by COVID-19 patients in the North is statistically significantly higher than in the rest of England, even after accounting for age, ethnicity, deprivation, and health conditions. In these first 12 months of the pandemic, the adjusted percentage of hospital beds occupied by COVID-19 patients in the North is: 1.0 percentage point more in the North compared to the rest of England, including London (95% CI: 1.0 to 1.1). This is equivalent to 10 per cent more hospital beds occupied by COVID-19 patients in the North than in the rest of England.

This increased pressure on hospitals in the North is also reflected in terms of disproportionate decreases in other hospital activity during the COVID-19 pandemic. Data from the Institute for Fiscal Studies (Burn et al, 2021) has found that between March and December 2020, there were 2.9 million (34 per cent) fewer elective (planned) inpatient admissions, 1.2 million (21 per cent) fewer non-COVID-19 emergency inpatient admissions, and 17.1 million (22 per cent) fewer outpatient appointments compared with the same period in 2019. They additionally found that these reductions were not uniformly spread across the country, with some regions seeing larger reductions than others. In general, the Northern regions experienced larger reductions than the national average (with the exception of the North East for emergency inpatient procedures).

Specifically, for elective inpatient procedures: Yorkshire and The Humber experienced a 5 percentage point (or 14.5 per cent) larger reduction than the national average; the North West experienced a two percentage point (or 5.8 per cent) larger reduction than the national average; and the North East experienced a 1.5 percentage point (or 4.3 per cent) larger reduction than the national average. For emergency inpatient procedures: Yorkshire and The Humber experienced a 2.7 percentage point (or 12.7 per cent) larger reduction than the national average; the North West experienced a 2 percentage point (or 9.4 per cent) larger reduction than the national average; and the North East experienced a 0.5 percentage point (or 2.4 per cent) smaller reduction than the national average. For outpatient procedures: Yorkshire and The Humber experienced a 2.1 percentage point (or 9.6 per cent) larger reduction than the national average; the North West experienced a 1.2 percentage point (or 5.5 per cent) larger reduction than the national average; and the North East experienced a 0.6 percentage point (or 2.8 per cent) larger reduction than the national average. These additional pressures may have long-term impacts on the availability of health care in the North for years 'after' the pandemic.

Regional trends in long COVID

It is now established that a range of symptoms can remain long after acute COVID-19 infection: long COVID. The official NHS guidelines on managing the long-term effects of COVID-19 define long COVID as ongoing symptoms of COVID-19 that persist beyond four weeks from initial infection (NICE, 2020). Studies have shown that long COVID impacts on multiple organs and can affect many systems including, but not limited to, the respiratory, cardiovascular, neurological, gastrointestinal, and musculoskeletal systems (Crook et al, 2021). The main symptoms of long COVID include fatigue, shortness of breath, cardiac problems, cognitive impairment and concentration problems (brain fog), stroke, gastrointestinal problems, insomnia, depression, anxiety muscle pain, and headache (among others).

Survey data from the ONS on the prevalence of long COVID in the UK for June 2022 estimated that around 1.6 million people (three per cent of the population) were experiencing self-reported long COVID.[19] Of these, around eight in ten (81 per cent) reported experiencing long COVID symptoms at least 12 weeks after first having (suspected) COVID-19, around four in ten (43 per cent) at least one year after, and around two in ten (21 per cent) at least two years after (ONS, 2022). The most common long COVID symptoms were fatigue (54 per cent), shortness of breath (31 per cent), loss of smell (23 per cent), and muscle ache (22 per cent). Self-reported long COVID was more common in: those aged 35 to 69 years, women, people living in more deprived areas, those working in social care, those aged 16–64 years who were not in or looking for paid work, and those with another activity-limiting health condition or disability.[20]

Using this data, we calculated there are also regional inequalities in long COVID (Table 3.2): 3.7 per cent of the population in the North had long COVID of any duration compared to 2.8 in the rest of England; long COVID of at least four weeks' duration was estimated to affect 2.8 per cent of people living in the North, compared to 2.1 per cent in the rest of England; and for at least 12 months' duration, the prevalence rates were respectively 1.6 per cent and 1.2 per cent for the North and the rest of the country. Long COVID rates of any duration ranged from 4.2 per cent in the North East to 2.2 per cent in London, with a national average of 2.8 per cent. Given that long COVID symptoms adversely affected the day-to-day activities of 72 per cent of people in the sample, this greater long-term morbidity in the North could have significant impacts on the lives and livelihoods of the population – potentially increasing regional social and economic inequalities into the future.

Table 3.2: Prevalence of long COVID by region: population estimate (in thousands) and percentage of population with long COVID (of any duration, at least 12 weeks' duration, at least 12 months' duration), June 2022

	N any duration	% any duration	N 12 weeks duration	% 12 weeks duration	N 12 months duration	% 12 months duration
North East	107	4.2	82	3.2	47	1.8
North West	250	3.5	190	2.7	105	1.5
Yorkshire and The Humber	179	3.4	134	2.5	73	1.4
East Midlands	138	3.0	101	2.2	60	1.3
West Midlands	162	2.8	118	2.1	59	1.0
East of England	184	3.0	140	2.3	78	1.3
London	192	2.2	142	1.6	89	1.0
South East	263	3.0	192	2.2	114	1.3
South West	169	3.1	112	2.0	60	1.1
North	536	3.7	406	2.8	225	1.6
Rest of England	1,108	2.8	805	2.1	460	1.2
England	1,644	3.0	1,211	2.2	685	1.3

Source: Calculated from ONS (2022)

Conclusion

This chapter has examined regional trends in the 'parallel pandemics' of mental health, hospital pressure, and long

COVID. For all three areas we find disturbing trends for the North which do not bode well for future regional health inequalities. In terms of mental health during the COVID-19 pandemic, we found that, on average, both the North and the rest of England experienced a deterioration in mental health during the pandemic – but that this decline has been more sustained in the North. We also found that across England, women had worse average mental health scores than men and that people from an ethnic minority background had worse mental health than people from a White British background. This was particularly evident for ethnic minority women in the North. We found that the gap in average mental health scores between the lowest and highest household income groups grew over the pandemic and remains large. Finally, we found that young adults in the North suffered the largest increase in probable non-psychotic mental illness. Our findings for self-reported mental health were supported by our analysis of anti-depressant prescribing which found that the North experienced greater rates of anti-depressant prescriptions per person – both before and during the pandemic. This chapter has also presented evidence that the North was hit the hardest in terms of hospital bed occupancy due to COVID-19. It also experienced larger reductions in elective inpatient, emergency inpatient, and outpatient procedures. We also found that long COVID rates are significantly higher in the Northern regions. The unequal nature of these 'parallel pandemics' could lead to an increase in morbidity in the North over the longer term alongside reductions in access to health care. In the next chapter we discuss the broader economic impacts of COVID-19 and estimate the cost of these unequal health impacts on the North specifically.

FOUR

The costs of COVID-19: regional economic inequalities

Introduction

This chapter examines the regional impact of the COVID-19 economic crisis. Through analysing official data we examine regional trends in lockdowns, unemployment rates, furlough rates, and wage levels. We will also calculate the productivity costs to the UK economy of the higher COVID-19 mortality (Chapter Two) and mental health morbidity (Chapter Three) experienced in the North. We find that the North, again, was disproportionately affected. On average, people living in the North spent longer in the most restrictive lockdown tiers, were more likely to become unemployed, and saw their wages fall. We conservatively estimate that the disproportionate health effects of the pandemic on the North could cost the UK economy over £9 billion per year.

Lockdowns

On the 23 March 2020 the government announced the first national lockdown, which would remain in place until 4 July 2020 ('Freedom Day') when the rules were significantly eased. The second national lockdown was introduced from 5 November 2020 until 2 December 2020 and the third was from 6 January 2021 through to 12 April 2021. With the introduction of the initial lockdown in March 2020, the rules set out required everyone to 'stay at home', with allowances to leave their homes for: shopping for basic necessities, one form of exercise a day, any medical needs, to provide care or help to vulnerable persons and travelling to and from work if necessary. Non-essential shops, gyms, and schools were closed. The second national lockdown saw similar restrictions while during the third one, schools remained open.

Outside the periods of a national lockdown, areas with a high number of COVID-19 cases were assessed and local lockdown restrictions were applied. The level of restrictions were relative to the rise of COVID-19 cases and were more formally applied from 14 October 2020 until 5 January 2021, with local authorities assigned to one of four different alert levels (with Level 4 being the most restrictive – see Box 4.1).

The local lockdowns meant that there were differing levels of lockdown restrictions across the country. To explore the differences, we retrospectively applied the tiered approach that came into force in October 2020 to assign a lockdown level to each local authority. We used data available from government briefings to assign a lockdown level to each day from the 23 March 2020 to the 12 April 2021.

Across the period of the pandemic, where a national lockdown was not in place, the North experienced greater levels in higher tiers of lockdown (Figure 4.1). In particular, during the summer months of July 2020 to September 2020 the North was in a higher level of lockdown.

Regionally, on average, people in the North West experienced the fewest number of days in the lowest tier of lockdown, Tier 1 (87.5 days; 22.7 per cent) (Figure 4.2, panel a). For the mean number of days in Tier 2, people in the North East (54.0 days; 14.0 per cent) and the North West (69.5 days; 18.0 per cent) experienced the least and second least number

Box 4.1: Local lockdown tiers in England

Level One – medium alert:

- meetings of groups up to six people indoor or outdoor
- travel to be limited
- all shops to open including the hospitality sector
- gyms and leisure facilities to open
- sporting events to open to public with a maximum capacity of 4000 outdoors or 2000 indoors.

Level Two – high alert:

- meetings of groups up to six people outdoor and only indoor if within support bubble
- travel but avoiding travel to areas in other tiers
- all shops to open, including the hospitality sector only if a substantial meal is served
- gyms and leisure facilities to open
- sporting events to open to public with a maximum capacity of 2000 outdoors or 1000 indoors.

Level Three – very high alert:

- only meeting with those in support bubble
- no travel outside area
- shops to open but the hospitality sector closed
- gyms and leisure facilities to open.

Level Four – stay at home:

- stay at home as much as possible and not meet others
- no travel
- only essential shops open.

of days, respectively. In contrast, people in the North West and North East experienced the most number of days in very high alert, tier three (77.3 days; 20.0 per cent, and 67.3 days; 17.4 per cent respectively). People in the North West experienced the most number of days in the highest level of lockdown, tier four (151.7 days; 39.3 per cent).

Figure 4.1: Mean lockdown level by month between the North and the rest of England

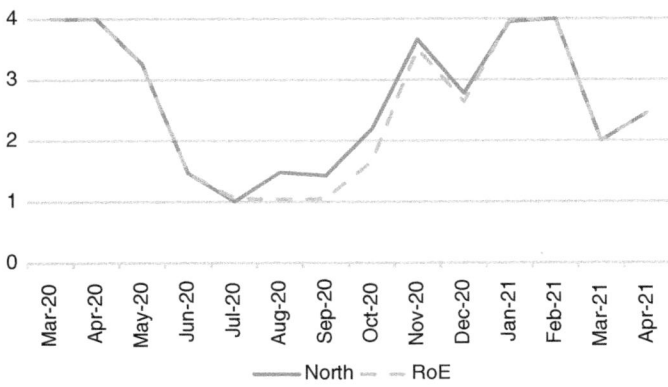

Note: Level 1 = medium alert; Level 2 = high alert; Level 3 = very high alert; Level 4 = stay at home

When comparing those in the North to the rest of England, we see that a higher percentage of days were spent in higher levels of lockdown (Figure 4.2). People in the North spent 54.6 per cent of the time in the two most restrictive tiers of lockdowns, compared to 46.3 per cent in the rest of the country. This means that, on average, people in the North had 41 more days (almost six weeks) of the harshest restrictions than people in the rest of the country. This was even worse in the North West, which spent 59.3 per cent of the time under the strictest lockdown, compared to 41.1 per cent in the South West. People in the North West therefore had 70 more days (ten weeks) in the top two tiers.

Economic impacts

Here we examine regional inequalities in the economic impacts of the pandemic. In particular, we focus on differences between the North and the rest of England in terms of unemployment, furlough, and wages. These are important

Figure 4.2: Percentage of time spent in each tier of lockdown

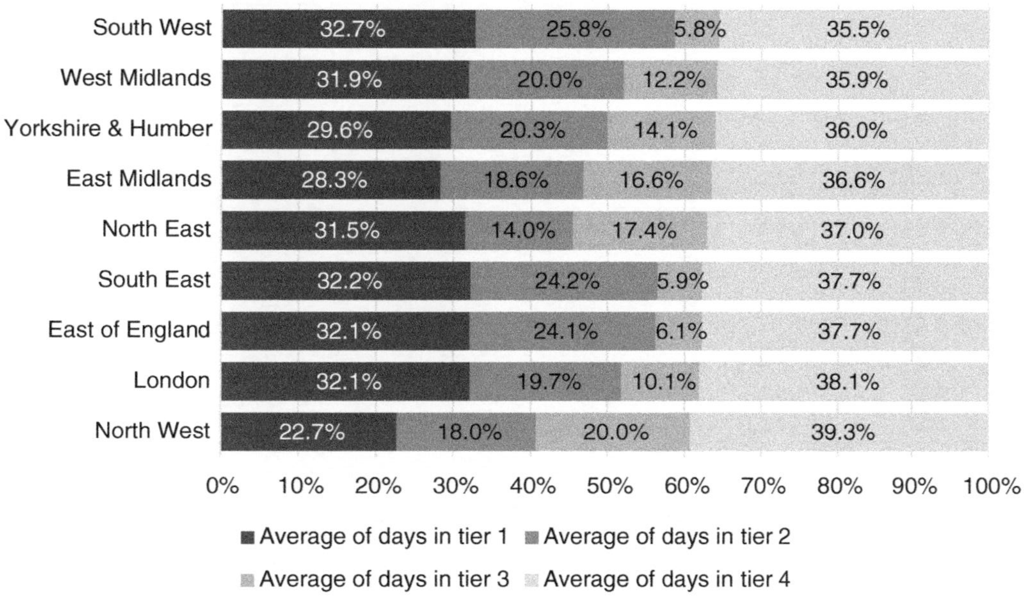

Region	Average of days in tier 1	Average of days in tier 2	Average of days in tier 3	Average of days in tier 4
South West	32.7%	25.8%	5.8%	35.5%
West Midlands	31.9%	20.0%	12.2%	35.9%
Yorkshire & Humber	29.6%	20.3%	14.1%	36.0%
East Midlands	28.3%	18.6%	16.6%	36.6%
North East	31.5%	14.0%	17.4%	37.0%
South East	32.2%	24.2%	5.9%	37.7%
East of England	32.1%	24.1%	6.1%	37.7%
London	32.1%	19.7%	10.1%	38.1%
North West	22.7%	18.0%	20.0%	39.3%

■ Average of days in tier 1   ■ Average of days in tier 2
■ Average of days in tier 3   ▨ Average of days in tier 4

Note: Tier 1 is the lowest level of restrictions and Tier 4 is the highest level of restrictions.

Figure 4.3: Mean unemployment rate (per cent) across a 14 month period of COVID-19 pandemic (March 2020 to April 2021) by region

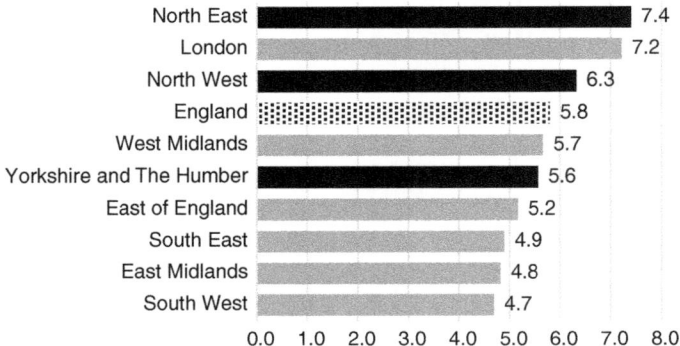

Note: The three regions in the North are coloured black. The remaining nine regions in the rest of England are coloured grey. The English average is shown as a hashed bar.

outcomes in their own right but are also key social determinants of health. We show that the North experienced higher rates of unemployment and reductions in wages but lower rates of furloughed employments during the COVID-19 pandemic compared to the rest of England.

Unemployment rates

COVID-19 affected many aspects of people's lives, including employment opportunities. To investigate how COVID-19 has impacted these areas, we use data on the local authority unemployment claimant count, published by the ONS, as a proxy for unemployment rates.[1] The mean claimant count rates across the first 14 months of the pandemic (March 2020 to April 2021) are shown in Figure 4.3. The North East and the North West experienced the highest (7.4 per cent) and third highest claimant count (6.3 per cent), respectively. Yorkshire and The Humber experienced the fifth highest claimant count (5.6 per cent). The South West and East Midlands had the lowest (4.7 per cent) and second lowest (4.8 per cent) claimant count, respectively.

Figure 4.4: The North vs rest of England time trend of unemployment rate (per cent) between March 2020 and March 2021

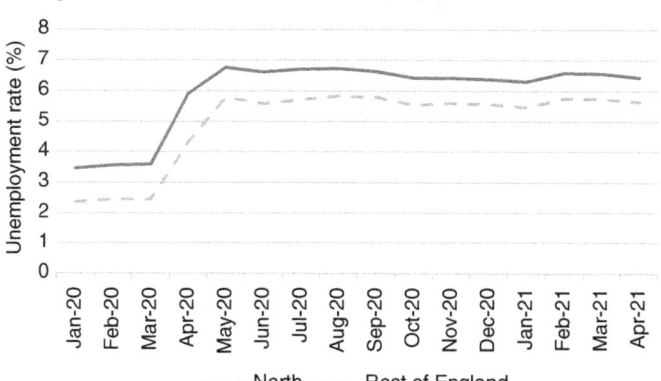

Figure 4.4 shows that the North, on average, had higher unemployment rates than the rest of the country throughout the duration of the pandemic (Munford et al, 2021).

To examine if there were differential effects of the unemployment outcomes in the North compared to the rest of England, we used models 1 to 4 from Chapter 2. The outcome measure in these models is the mean claimant count during the pandemic (March 2020 to April 2021). We also adjusted for other factors (age, ethnicity, and deprivation). During the first 14 months of the pandemic, the unemployment rate in the North was significantly higher than in the rest of England.

In the unadjusted model (Model 1), the unemployment rate in the North (6.3 per cent) was an additional one percentage point higher (95% CI: 0.49 to 1.40) compared to the rest of England (5.3 per cent). In relative terms, the unemployment rate in the North was 19 per cent higher than in the rest of England, on average, during the first 14 months of the pandemic. Even after accounting for age, ethnicity, and deprivation (Model 4), unemployment rates were 0.35 percentage points higher in the North compared to the rest of England.

Figure 4.5: Mean furlough uptake rates across 11 month period (May 2020 to March 2021) by region

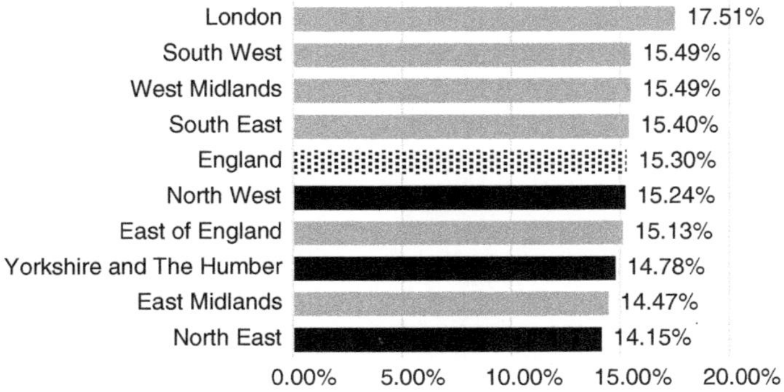

Furlough uptake

In late March 2020, the government announced that they would introduce a furlough scheme to help mitigate against the threat of mass unemployment. This scheme enabled employers to temporarily stop paying their workforce and the government would pay 80 per cent of their usual wage.[2] However, this was only in effect for national lockdowns – not local ones. We used furlough uptake data from the Job Retention Scheme Statistics to investigate the regional inequalities in furlough rates.[3]

Figure 4.5 shows the variability in the average furlough rates by region between the months of May 2020 and April 2021. Across the 11 month period the North East (14.2 per cent), Yorkshire and The Humber (14.8 per cent), and the North West (15.2 per cent) had the lowest, third, and fifth lowest furlough rates. Over the whole time period, on average there was very little difference between the North and the rest of England.[4]

Wages

We obtained information on weekly gross pay from NOMIS in 2019 and 2020.[5] Figure 4.6 plots this data for the three

Figure 4.6: Median pay in 2019 and 2020, by area

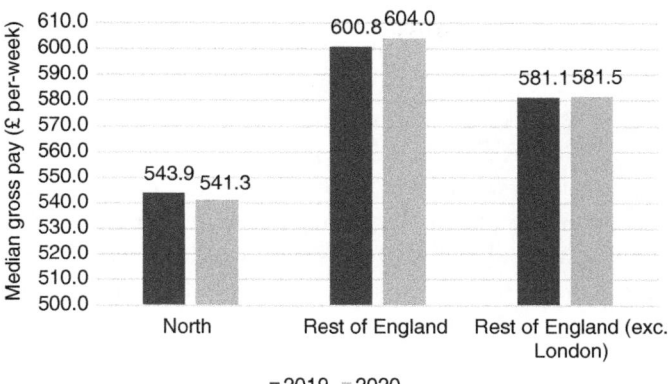

regional configurations: the North, the rest of England and the rest of England (excluding London).[6] It is clear that wages in the North, on average, are much lower than the rest of the country, even when London is excluded. Also, during the pandemic wages in the North fell slightly (from £543.9 to £541.3 per week) whereas they very slightly increased in the rest of the country (from £600.80 to £604.00).

The pandemic and productivity

The effect of higher COVID deaths in the North on productivity

As noted in Chapter One, in 2018 we published a report with the Northern Health Science Alliance called *Health for Wealth* (Bambra et al, 2018). This demonstrated that before the pandemic around 30 per cent of the £4 per hour productivity gap between the North and the rest of England was attributable to poorer health in the North. This 30 per cent figure was comprised of 17.1 per cent attributable to higher morbidity (ill-health) and 12.8 per cent attributable to higher mortality.[7] In this report, the unadjusted difference in all-cause mortality (per-year) between the North and the rest of England was 112 extra deaths per 100,000 population per year. During the first year of the pandemic, the unadjusted difference in all-cause mortality between the North and the rest of England (including London, to be consistent) was an extra 145.8 deaths per 100,000 population (Munford et al, 2021). So, assuming linearity, if an additional 112 deaths per 100,000 population contributed 12.8 per cent to the productivity gap, it can be inferred that an additional 145.8 deaths per 100,000 population will contribute 16.7 per cent to the regional productivity gap. Further, 16.7 per cent of the productivity gap (of £44 billion) between the North and the rest of England equates to a potential loss of £7.3 billion in GDP brought about by unequal mortality rates in the North and the rest of England. This figure is likely to be an underestimate, however, and should be re-evaluated at the end of the pandemic and in light of other trends such as the 2022 cost of living crisis as these other macroeconomic factors are likely to further exacerbate the gap in productivity between the North and the rest of England.

Impact of higher rates of mental ill health on productivity

As noted in previous sections of this chapter, during the pandemic, productivity has fallen throughout the country for a number of reasons, including unemployment and furlough. Previously in this chapter, we demonstrated that this has not been equally spread across England, and the North has, on average, fared worse. We have additionally previously demonstrated that health is important for productivity too (Bambra et al, 2018). Given the huge mental health impacts of the pandemic on the North (Chapter Three), we expect the parallel pandemic of mental ill health to further negatively affect the regional productivity gap. In Chapter Three, we observed that the pandemic had caused a decline in mental health across the country – but particularly in the North. During the pandemic, mental health (as measured by the 12 item General Health Questionnaire, GHQ-12) fell by 0.5 points in North (equivalent to 8.87 per cent of a standard deviation).

Here, we use past estimates of the relationship between reductions in mental health and economic productivity to estimate the potential cost to the economy of this reduction in mental health in the North. Using data from 2011 to 2018 (latest available data), we ran a fixed-effects linear model to estimate the relationship between mental wellbeing (measured using the Small Area Mental Health Index [SAMHI], a composite measure of mental health)[8] and GVA[9] at a local authority level within the North.[10] We also accounted for population characteristics known to be associated with GVA (including education and ethnicity). The results from this model are presented in Figure 4.7, where it can be seen that a one standard deviation increase in poor mental wellbeing was associated with a £1,491 decrease in GVA per-head in the North.[11]

Given that COVID-19 caused an 8.87 per cent (of a standard deviation) decrease in mental health in the North, we estimate this could translate into around a £132 per person (= 0.0887 × £1491) reduction in GVA per-head in the North. Given a population size of 15.5 million people in the North, this loss in GVA in the study period is equivalent to around £2 billion (£2,046,000,000) in the period April 2020 to September 2021. This is shown in Figure 4.7 and Table 4.1.

Productivity has fallen during the pandemic because of economic factors including unemployment and furlough. However, we know that health – in particular mental health – also affects productivity. We have shown here that the effects of the pandemic on mental health within the North of England could costs the UK economy an additional £2 billion.

Figure 4.7: The relationship between mental health and gross value added (GVA) at local authority level within the North, 2011–2018

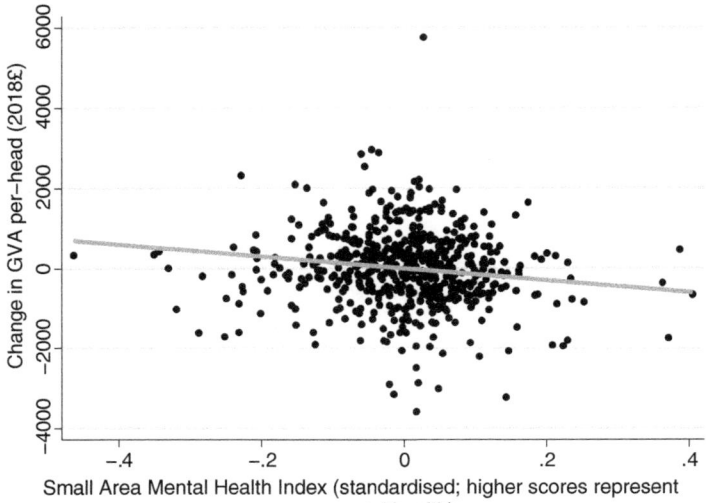

Small Area Mental Health Index (standardised; higher scores represent worse mental health)

Note: Fixed–effects regression; 2011–2018. Coef. = –1491.84, se = 410.45, t = –3.63. The model also includes year fixed-effects, the LAD's total population (number of people), the per cent of the population (aged over 16+) who have no qualifications, the per cent of the population (aged over 16+) who are aged 16–64, and the per cent of the population (aged over 16+) who are white UK nationals. GVA is deflated to 2018 prices. The regression was weighted by the size of the LAD population. Full regression results are contained in Table 4.1.

Conclusion

This chapter has examined regional differences on the impact that COVID-19 had on economic outcomes, including lockdowns, unemployment, furlough, and wages. It then estimated the potential costs to future economic productivity caused by the unequal effects of the pandemic on mortality and mental health. We found that, in terms of lockdowns, the North of England spent much longer in the more restrictive

Table 4.1: The relationship between mental health and gross value added (GVA) per head at local authority level within the North, 2011–2018

	GVA per-head (2018 £)
SAMHI	−1491.839***
	(−2298.310 to −685.368)
Population size (number of people)	−0.018
	(−0.038 to 0.002)
% of population (aged 16+) with no qualifications	−12.785
	(−64.648 to 39.078)
% of population (aged 16+) who are aged 16–64	−15.881
	(−85.487 to 53.725)
% of population (aged 16+) who are white UK nationals	21.129
	(−33.143 to 75.401)
Year effects (base=2011)	
2012	370.746*
	(28.230 to 713.263)
2013	637.368**
	(254.928 to 1019.808)
2014	1150.600***
	(671.811 to 1629.389)
2015	1901.077***
	(1353.403 to 2448.752)
2016	2160.251***
	(1524.909 to 2795.593)
2017	2602.668***
	(1893.408 to 3311.927)

(continued)

Table 4.1: The relationship between mental health and GVA per head at local authority level within the North, 2011–2018 (continued)

2018	3069.439***
	(2227.608 to 3911.270)
N	72
Observations (N*T)	569

Note: Model is a fixed-effects linear model to account for within LAD variation. The model is additionally weighted by the population size of a LAD. SAMHI = small-area mental health index, standardised to have mean zero and unitary standard deviation. It is increasing in poor mental health (higher scores relate to worse mental health outcomes). GVA is deflated to 2018 prices. 95% confidence intervals in brackets. * $p < 0.05$; ** $p < 0.01$; *** $p < 0.001$.

tiers of lockdown restrictions than the rest of England. These lockdowns limited people's movements and hence reduced their social interactions but also their economic activities. There was considerably higher unemployment in the North of England throughout the pandemic, increasing the employment gap between the North and the rest of England. Employment is a key social determinant of health, and hence regional health inequalities could grow in the future. There was no evidence of regional differences furlough uptake, potentially because the North had higher unemployment rates instead and perhaps because furlough was not available during local lockdowns. Those who remained in employment in the North saw their pay slightly decrease between 2019 and 2020 while workers in the rest of England saw a slight increase. Finally, we conservatively estimate that the unequal health impacts of the pandemic on the North could cost the UK economy around £9.3 billion per-year in lost economic productivity (£7.3 billion from increased excess Northern mortality plus £2 billion from worse mental health in the North). Taken together, this chapter paints a worrying picture of the state of the Northern economy (and the UK economy as a whole). In the next chapter, we reflect on these findings alongside those of Chapters Two and Three in terms of what may have caused the unequal economic, mortality and morbidity impacts of the pandemic.

FIVE

Perfect storm: understanding the North–South pandemic divide

Our analysis has found that the COVID-19 pandemic was a regionally unequal pandemic: deaths from COVID-19 were 17 per cent higher in the North (29.4 more deaths per 100,000); mental health declines were more sustained in the North; hospital pressures were 10 per cent higher during the pandemic in the North; the morbidity burden of long COVID is 30 per cent higher in the North; and the economic impacts have been deeper – potentially costing the Northern economy £9 billion in lost productivity. This discussion chapter seeks to understand these results by placing them within the wider conceptual and empirical context of the health and place literature as set out in the introductory Chapter One. Using the syndemic pandemic, deprivation amplification, and intersectionality concepts and drawing on the political economy of health approach, it explores how the regional inequalities in health and wealth we have identified during the pandemic reflect longer-term divides within the country.

The syndemic pandemic

We have shown that deaths from COVID-19 were 17 per cent higher in the North (Chapter Two). As noted in the introductory Chapter One, the North was left more exposed to the adverse impacts of the pandemic because of decades of long-term economic – and health – decline. The COVID-19 pandemic occurred against a backdrop of large social and economic regional inequalities in non-communicable diseases (NCDs) as well as inequalities in the social determinants of health. Inequalities in COVID-19 therefore arose because of a syndemic of COVID-19, inequalities in chronic diseases, and the social determinants of health (Figure 5.1). The prevalence and severity of the COVID-19 pandemic was magnified in the North because of the pre-existing epidemics of chronic disease and deprivation – which are themselves socially patterned and associated with the social determinants of health (Smith et al, 2016). This meant that the population in the North was less resilient and less prepared for the COVID-19 pandemic: a perfect storm of inequality and infection.

The higher rates of deprivation and long-term health conditions in the North are leading factors in any explanation of why the North fared worse in terms of COVID-19 deaths and ill health. In previous work, we have outlined that for more deprived communities – predominantly located in the North, COVID-19 was experienced as a 'syndemic pandemic' – whereby COVID-19 interacted with – and exacerbated – pre-existing social, economic, and health inequalities (Bambra et al, 2020a, 2021a).[1, 2] The concept of a syndemic was developed by the anthropologist and clinician Dr Merrill Singer (2000; 2009) in his work examining the synergistic nature of the epidemics of HIV/AIDS, substance use, and violence in the US in the 1990s. A syndemic exists when risk factors or co-morbidities are intertwined, interactive, and cumulative – that is, when multiple causes of ill health pile upon and reinforce each other in ways that

Figure 5.1: The syndemic of COVID-19, non-communicable diseases (NCDs) and the social determinants of health

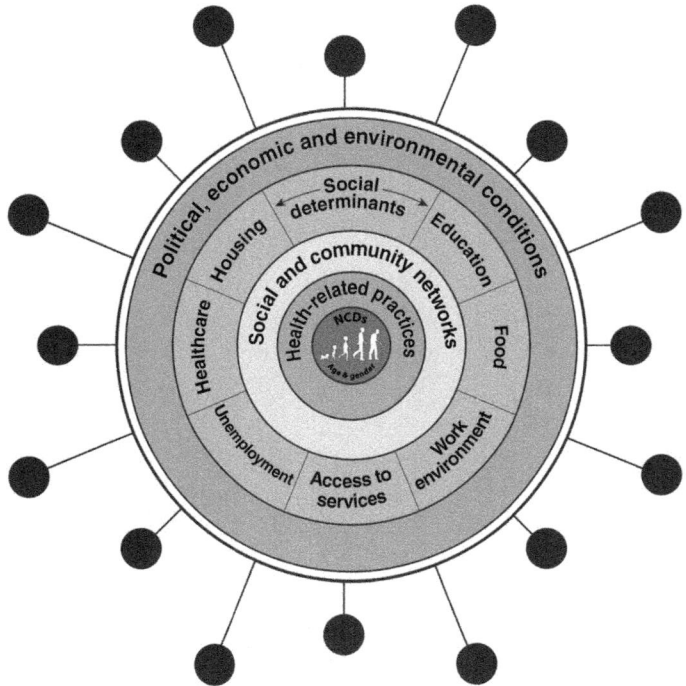

Source: Reproduced under Commons Creative Licence from Bambra et al (2020a)

make illness from COVID-19 more common and more damaging: 'A syndemic is a set of closely intertwined and mutual enhancing health problems that significantly affect the overall health status of a population within the context of a perpetuating configuration of noxious social conditions' (Singer, 2000: 9). For the most disadvantaged communities, COVID-19 was experienced as a syndemic – a co-occurring, synergistic pandemic which interacts with and exacerbates existing inequalities in economic, social and health conditions (Figure 5.1).

Figure 5.2: Pathways to inequalities in COVID-19

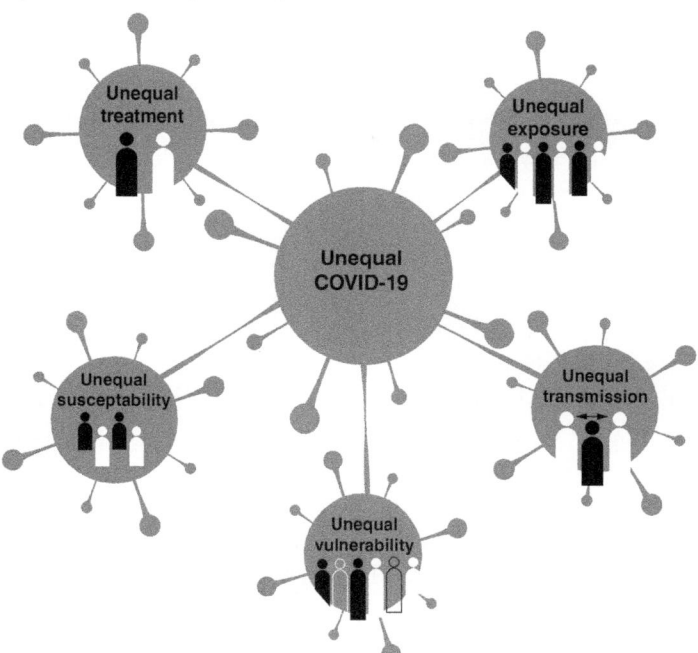

Source: Reproduced under Commons Creative Licence from Bambra (2021b)

Building on this, we have previously suggested that there are five potential pathways through which existing inequalities in the social determinants of health resulted in higher COVID-19 mortality and morbidity: unequal exposure, transmission, vulnerability, susceptibility, and treatment (Figure 5.2):

- *Unequal exposure*: These inequalities in chronic conditions arise as a result of inequalities in exposure to the social determinants of health: the conditions in which people 'live, work, grow and age' including working conditions, unemployment, access to essential goods and services (for example water, sanitation and food), housing, and access to health care (WHO, 2008; Dahlgren and Whitehead, 1991). By way of example, there are considerable occupational inequalities in exposure to adverse working conditions (for example ergonomic hazards, repetitive work, long hours, shift work, low wages, job insecurity) – they are concentrated in lower skill jobs. These working conditions are associated with increased risks of respiratory diseases, certain cancers, musculoskeletal disease, hypertension, stress, and anxiety (Bambra, 2011). In addition to these long-term exposures, inequalities in working conditions may well be impacting on the unequal distribution of the COVID-19 disease burden. For example, lower paid workers – particularly in the service sector (such as food, cleaning or delivery services) – were less likely to be able to work from home – and much more likely to be designated as key workers and thereby still required to go into work, even during lockdowns. They were also much more likely to be reliant on public transport for doing so. Insecure work and lack of sick pay from employers and the state also reduces the ability for these workers to self-isolate when symptomatic. These all increase exposure to the virus.

- *Unequal transmission*: Inequalities in housing conditions may also be contributing to inequalities in COVID-19. Housing is also an important factor in driving health inequalities (Gibson et al, 2011). For example, exposure to poor quality housing is associated with certain health outcomes (damp housing can lead to respiratory diseases such as asthma while overcrowding can result in higher infection rates and increased risk of injury from household accidents). Overcrowding and less spacious housing is associated with higher C-reactive protein levels, a biomarker of inflammation and stress (Clair and Hughes, 2019). Housing also impacts health inequalities materially through costs (for example as a result of high rents) and psychosocially through insecurity (for example short-term leases). More deprived communities have a higher exposure to poor quality, unaffordable, or insecure housing, and therefore have a higher rate of negative health consequences (McNamara et al, 2017). These inequalities in housing conditions may also contribute to inequalities in COVID-19. For example, deprived neighbourhoods are more likely to contain houses of multiple occupation, smaller houses with a lack of outside space, as well as have higher population densities (particularly in deprived urban areas) and lower access to communal green space (Bambra, 2016). These will likely increase COVID-19 transmission (and therefore mortality) rates – as was the case with H1N1, where strong associations were found with urbanity (Rutter et al, 2012).

- *Unequal vulnerability*: A higher burden of pre-existing health conditions (such as diabetes and respiratory conditions, heart disease, obesity) increases the severity and mortality of COVID-19. People living in areas of higher deprivation generally have a greater number of co-existing chronic health conditions, which are more severe, and they experience them at a younger age. Research has shown that chronic conditions – such as hypertension, diabetes, asthma, COPD, heart, liver, and renal disease, cancer, cardiovascular disease, obesity and smoking – increase the likelihood of complications and deaths due to COVID-19 (Bambra et al, 2020a). For example, people with diabetes are three times more likely to experience severe symptoms of death from COVID-19, smokers are 1.5 times more likely to experience severe symptoms and the odds of developing severe COVID-19 are up to seven times higher in patients with obesity (Alqahtani et al, 2020; Roncon et al, 2020; Simonnet et al, 2020). People living in more disadvantaged neighbourhoods have higher rates of almost all of these known underlying clinical risk factors that increase the severity of and death from COVID-19 (Guo et al, 2019).

- *Unequal susceptibility*: The social determinants of health also work to make people from marginalised communities more vulnerable to infection from COVID-19 – even when they have no underlying health conditions. Decades of research into the psychosocial determinants of health have found that the chronic stresses of material and psychological deprivation are associated with immunosuppression (Segerstrom and Miller, 2004). Psychosocial feelings of subordination or inferiority as a result of occupying a low position on the social hierarchy stimulate physiological stress responses (for example raised cortisol levels) which, when prolonged (chronic), can have long-term adverse consequences for physical and mental health (Bartley, 2016). By way of example, studies have found consistent associations between low job status (for example low control and high demands), stress-related morbidity, and various chronic conditions, including coronary heart disease, hypertension, obesity, musculoskeletal conditions, and psychological ill health (Bambra, 2011). Likewise, there is increasing evidence that living in disadvantaged environments may produce a sense of powerlessness and collective threat among residents leading to chronic stressors that, in time, damage health (Whitehead et al, 2016). Studies have also confirmed that adverse psychosocial circumstances increase susceptibility – influencing the onset, course, and outcome of infectious diseases – including respiratory diseases like COVID-19 (Biondi et al, 1997).

- *Unequal treatment*: Similarly, access to health care is lower in disadvantaged and marginalised communities – even in universal health care systems (Todd et al, 2015). In England, the number of patients per general practitioner is 15 per cent higher in the most deprived areas than in least deprived (Lacobucci, 2019). This reduced access to health care – before and during the outbreak – contributes to inequalities in chronic disease and is also likely to lead to worse outcomes from COVID-19 in more disadvantaged areas and marginalised communities. Further, because of health services having to focus on combating the pandemic, there has also been a significant reduction in health care access for people with existing chronic conditions such as cancer or cardiovascular disease. Similarly, access to preventative care has also been restricted because of health care system pressures and the need for social distancing. This will also likely disproportionately impact on populations with higher rates of NCDs – such as the North. Since the vaccine rollout programme, there has also been emerging evidence of higher rates of vaccine hesitancy and lower uptake in more deprived communities (Goffe et al, 2021; Todd and Bambra, 2021).

In related work, we have empirically tested the contribution of the first four of these pathways (exposure, transmission, vulnerability, susceptibility) to explaining the deprivation gap in COVID-19 deaths during the first wave of the pandemic (January to July 2020) in England (Albani et al, 2022). We used decomposition methods to explicitly quantify the independent contribution of four of the inequality pathways (exposure, transmission, vulnerability, susceptibility) in explaining the more severe COVID-19 outcomes in 205 of the most deprived local authorities compared to the rest. We found that inequalities in transmission (73 per cent) and in vulnerability (49 per cent) explained the highest proportion of mortality by deprivation (Figure 5.3). Given that the vast majority of the most deprived local authorities are located in the Northern regions, these links between deprivation and COVID-19 outcomes may well explain why the North fared so poorly in the pandemic: it has considerably higher rates of deprivation and underlying ill health than the rest of the country (as shown in Figure 1.6, Chapter 1).

Deprivation amplification

However, as our results in Chapters Two and Three show, the North was more adversely impacted by COVID-19 than

Figure 5.3: Visualisation of decomposition results: percentage of area-level deprivation gap in COVID-19 mortality explained by different pathways

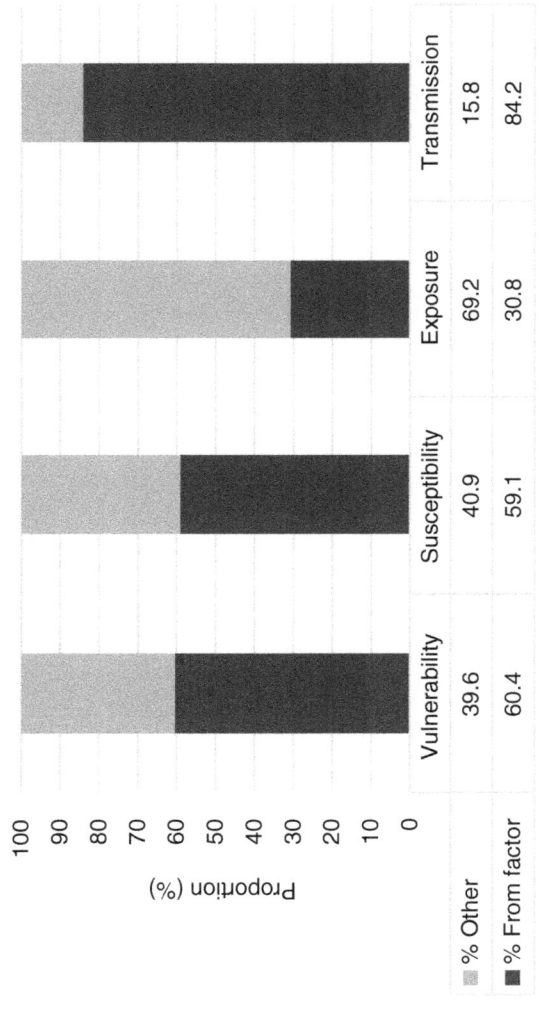

	Vulnerability	Susceptibility	Exposure	Transmission
% Other	39.6	40.9	69.2	15.8
% From factor	60.4	59.1	30.8	84.2

■ % From factor   ■ % Other

Source: Reproduced under Commons Creative Licence from Albani et al (2022)

would be expected based on deprivation alone. As such, the impacts of deprivation were 'amplified' in the North both for COVID-19 outcomes and in terms of mental health and hospital pressures.

The concept of deprivation amplification (Chapter One) is potentially relevant to thinking about such influences. The deprivation amplification theory draws on the wider health geography literature on health and place – particularly the *context-composition-relational* debate (as outlined in Chapter One). Engaging with this debate, the deprivation amplification hypothesis asserts that the negative health effects of individual-level low SES (*composition*) are amplified (*relational*) for those living in more deprived areas (*context*) (Macintyre et al, 1993). In the literature, this concept has largely been applied to examining whether differential access to resources (context) between local areas impacts on the relationship between low SES (compositional) and health (Macintyre et al, 2008). Most notably this work has examined whether individual-level SES inequalities in physical activity are compounded by area-level characteristics (Macintyre, 2007; Schneider et al, 2019). In this regard, the concept of deprivation amplification has been subject to some debate. For example, some studies have found support for the thesis – that individual SES inequalities in physical activity are higher in more deprived areas (Macintyre et al, 2008) while others have not (Macintyre, 2007; Schneider et al, 2019).

Our results in Chapter Two find support for the thesis – suggesting that COVID-19 deaths in more deprived areas in the North were amplified. This may be because the syndemic pathways of inequality in COVID-19 can be exacerbated in areas of higher deprivation if they are embedded within a wider context of regional deprivation. Further, the deprivation amplification in the North may have resulted because of the more deep-seated and long-term nature of economic neglect in the North compared to the rest of England (as already noted in terms of declining life expectancy in the most deprived local authorities in the North compared to the rest of England in Figure 1.4 in Chapter One) – or because of nuances in Northern deprivation – as noted by the idea of Left Behind Areas. Left Behind Areas are defined as places that rank highly on the indices of multiple deprivation and lack key social infrastructure, including places and spaces to meet, connectivity (physical and digital), and community engagement (Munford et al, 2022b). There are 225 'left behind' neighbourhoods across England and these are predominantly located in post-industrial and coastal areas in the North (138 of 225 areas or 61 per cent). They have much worse socio-economic and health outcomes than the residents of other equally deprived areas (Munford et al, 2022b).

Placing intersectionality

The results from our analyses of self-reported mental health during the pandemic (Chapter Three) raise issues around the intersectional nature of health inequalities. We found that across the country, mental health declined during the COVID-19 pandemic, with scores at their lowest in January 2021. By September 2021, average mental health scores still had not returned to pre-pandemic levels. In our initial, unidimensional analyses, we found that before the pandemic, people from ethnic minority backgrounds had similar mental health scores to those from a White British background. However, at the start of the pandemic, people from ethnic minority backgrounds experienced a larger fall in mental health and this decline was greater for those from ethnic minority backgrounds in the North. Further, in our analyses assessing the intersection of sex, region and ethnicity, we found that ethnic minority women living in the North of England had the lowest average mental health scores throughout the pandemic. This raises important questions surrounding the potential processes shaping this inequality.

A growing body of research has discussed the possible reasons behind the high rates of COVID-19 in the ethnic minority populations of the UK. Arguably, many of the factors which disproportionately expose people from ethnic minority backgrounds to COVID-19 infection are many of the same factors which have affected the impact of the pandemic on their mental health. These include their disproportionate burden of chronic illness and co-morbidities, greater representation in the service economy and frontline health care roles, household overcrowding, and greater likelihood of residing in a deprived area (Lassale et al, 2020; Nguyen et al, 2020; Public Health England 2020b).

Another theory put forward relates to the 'ethnic density' hypothesis, whereby people from ethnic minority backgrounds have better health when they live in areas with a higher proportion of people from an ethnic minority background (Halpern and Nazroo, 1999). In a briefing note on COVID-19 and mental health by researchers at Understanding Society, it was observed that 'Pakistanis and Bangladeshis who live in areas with relatively high concentrations of own ethnic group residents have not experienced the same declines in mental health' (Nandi and Platt, 2020: 7). One of the pathways by which ethnic density is hypothesised to protect mental health is by improved local social support, social capital, and community cohesion (Bécares and Nazroo, 2013; Das-Munshi et al, 2010). The distribution of areas of high overall ethnic density is skewed towards the South of England. It is therefore possible that, compared to the North, the mental health of people from ethnic minority groups of people in the rest of the country was somehow protected by higher ethnic density during the pandemic.

An absence of additional social support and social capital offered by ethnic density may also have a disproportionate impact on women, as caring and home-schooling responsibilities were more likely to have fallen to women during the pandemic (Almeida et al, 2020). Women are also more likely to work in the service sector and in key worker roles than men, meaning they were more likely to still be required to work during the pandemic, but also likely did not have access to their usual childcare options (Blundell et al, 2022). Therefore, this is one possible theory behind the especially low average mental health scores for women from minority ethnic backgrounds in the North we observed in Figure 3.4.

Here we further reflect on the role that place (in our case region) plays in shaping these intersectional inequalities in mental health to understand why minority groups and young people in the North fared worse in terms of the parallel pandemic of mental health.

To date, the literature seeking to explain the relationship between health and place (Chapter One) has been dominated by the *composition-context* debate, its reconciliation via the relational (Cummings et al, 2007; Macintyre et al, 2002) and neo-materialist (Fox and Powell, 2021) perspectives, and, more recently, the integration of political economy and institutional perspectives (Bambra et al, 2019; Beckfield et al, 2015). However, despite the nuances in our theoretical understanding of the relationship between health and place that this evolution has provided, all the resulting research (from whichever perspective) has often been limited to the examination of the relationship between place, health, and a single axis of inequality (most notably area-level deprivation, and, to a lesser extent SES, ethnicity or migration [for example Bécares et al, 2013; Darlington-Pollock et al, 2017]) – with occasional reference to other factors such as gender (for example Rocha et al, 2017) or housing tenure (for example Darlington-Pollock and Norman, 2017). There has been little explicit integration into the geographies of health inequalities body of work of a more intersectional understanding of health inequalities and place – which explores how multiple axes of inequality are experienced simultaneously within – and as part of – a place (Evans, 2019a; 2019b or Bauer and Scheima, 2019).

The sizeable health inequalities literature has developed across quite independent streams but with a dominant (and arguably excluding) emphasis on socio-economic position (for example deprivation) as the key social determinant of health (Gkiouleka et al, 2018; Kapilashrami et al, 2015). Most health inequalities studies focus on single factors and mechanisms at a time – often even using single measures of SES (for example deprivation *or* occupation *or* income *or* education). Similarly, research into racial/ethnic health inequalities has often focused on the health disadvantage that members of minorities face due to their experience of interpersonal racism (Nazroo and Williams, 2005). Immigration has also been treated as a distinct category in health inequalities research (Krieger, 2000). Likewise, the gender and health inequalities literature has developed somewhat separately from the socio-economic and racial/ethnic literature (Bambra et al, 2021b). Sexuality and gender-identity research has also tended to be studied as autonomous from other dimensions of social difference (Gkiouleka et al, 2018).

This atomising approach in the health inequalities literature obscures the multiple stratification systems that people embody *simultaneously* (Krieger, 1997). The intersectional approach to health inequalities aims to address this by considering the cumulative, additive, and integrated nature of health inequalities and the converging processes associated with different categories of disadvantage (Graham et al, 2011). However, despite longstanding calls to integrate intersectionality analyses (Weber and Parra-Medina, 2003), it is only recently that health inequalities researchers have started to seriously undertake this process (see Evans, 2019a, 2019b or Bauer and Scheima, 2019). The intersectional inequalities in health literature are small.[3] Most notably, there has been very little integration of *place* itself as a facet of intersectionality in studies of health inequalities (with exception to recent work by Holman and colleagues. See: Holman et al, 2022). The geographical health inequalities literature (outlined in Chapter One) has also developed as an important (Gatrell and Elliot, 2009; Elliot, 2018), but distinct and separate body of work, seldom integrated into wider studies of health inequalities (Bambra, 2016). As a result, its insights are currently lacking in the emergent literature on intersectional health inequalities. So, just as analyses of health and place have been limited to the exploration of single axes of inequality, the potential role of place as an aspect of social location and identity – differentially shaping health outcomes for otherwise similar social groups – has been absent from intersectional research into health inequalities.

Our results in terms of the unequal impacts of the pandemic on mental health at the intersection of different social groups (age, gender, ethnicity) in different regions suggests that *place* shapes how these social categorisations were experienced during the pandemic. As such, *place* – and region specifically – should be considered as a crucial aspect of intersectionality (Hopkins, 2018). The results of other research examining the intersections of sexuality, class, race/ethnicity, age, and sexuality with location (for example Rodo´-de-Zarate, 2014; Schroeder, 2014) or exploring the intersectional nature of ethnic and religious identities, racism, gender, social class, and locality (Hopkins et al, 2017) reinforces our view. As Collins and Bilge (2016: 197) argue, 'social context has many interpretations' and they point to the importance of historic context, states, and their political and economic power, and social-cultural institutions as all contributing to 'social context' and localities. Indeed, Yuval-Davis (2015) describes intersectionality as a context-informed analytical tool that enables a focus on the social divisions shaping most people's lives (for example race and gender) and how this plays out in different contexts (for example time, place). So, our results on regional inequalities in mental health in different social groups during the pandemic suggest that the health and place literature needs to take a more explicitly intersectional approach, and the wider intersectionality and health inequalities field needs to consider the role that place plays as an aspect of intersectionality (Bambra, 2022a). So, we need to start to examine how social identities and their health implications play out differently across time, space, and place.

The political economy of health and wealth

The COVID-19 economic crisis – an economic shock of rare and extreme impact – had a devastating impact on the world economy with huge reductions in productivity, wages, and record levels of unemployment. Research from previous recessions suggests that the economic fallout from the COVID-19 pandemic might have a more negative – and a more sustained – impact on public health and health inequalities than the COVID-19 viral pandemic itself. In Chapter Four, we demonstrated that the UK COVID-19 emergency lockdowns had an unequal regional economic impact with the North faring worse with higher furlough and unemployment rates, and greater reductions in wages. We calculated that the productivity losses to the UK economy of the higher COVID-19 mortality (Chapter Two), mental health morbidity (Chapter Three) and the harsher lockdown restrictions experienced in the North amounted to £9 billion. As the economic impacts were unequal, previous research suggests that it is likely that the resulting health impacts will also be regionally unequal – exacerbating health inequalities. Here we draw on the political economy of health and place literature (Chapter One) to reflect on the health implications of the regionally unequal economic impacts of the pandemic.

National economic wealth (that is, GDP) has long been considered as the major global determinant of population health, with the vast differences in mortality between high- (for example UK, US, Europe) and low- and middle-income countries (for example India, Ethiopia, Ecuador) accounted for in terms of differences in economic growth (Freeman et al, 2020). Changes in the economy therefore potentially have important implications for population health and inequalities in health. Recessions are globally defined as two successive quarters of negative growth in GDP (Gamble, 2009). They are characterised by instability (in terms of inflation and interest rates) and sudden reductions in production and consumption with corresponding increases in business closures and unemployment. For example, the 'Global Financial Crisis' of 2007/8 was characterised by peaks in unemployment rates of around 8.5 per cent in the UK and the US, 10 per cent in France and more than 20 per cent in Spain.

The short-term overall population health effects of recessions are rather mixed with most international studies concluding that all-cause mortality, deaths from cardiovascular disease and from motor vehicle accidents, and hazardous health behaviours decrease during economic downturns, while deaths from suicides, rates of mental ill health and chronic illnesses increase (Bambra, 2011). Studies suggesting that recessions are 'good for health' have found that mortality rates rise during periods of economic growth (Gerdtham and Ruhm, 2006). For example, a study of mortality trends in the United States found that the overall decline in mortality rates in the 20th century reversed during periods of recession (Tapia Granados, 2005). One potential explanation of this inverse relationship between mortality rates and recession is that higher unemployment rates lead to a decrease in business activity and therefore a reduction in work-related deaths, combined with a reduction in alcohol and tobacco consumption as incomes reduce, resulting in a reduction in mortality risks (Adam, 1981). Studies have also found that road traffic accidents decrease during periods of recession, as people have less need to – and are less able to afford to – drive (Ruhm, 2000).

In contrast, in terms of mental illness, research also suggests that recessions can also be 'bad for health'. For instance, a study found that the mental health of men in England deteriorated over the two years following the Global Financial Crisis (Katikireddi et al, 2012). Mental health problems such as stress and depression were also found to increase during periods of recession in studies in Spain, Greece, and Northern Ireland (Economou et al, 2011; Houdmont et al, 2012; Gili et al, 2013). There is also evidence of increases in poor mental health and wellbeing after the Global Financial Crisis, including self-harm and psychiatric morbidity (Barnes et al, 2017; Vizard and Obolenskaya, 2015). In several studies this was found to lead to an increase in mortality rates during periods of recession, particularly from suicide (Barr et al, 2012). For example, following the 2007/8 crisis, worldwide an excess of 4884 suicides were observed in 2009 and over the next three years (2008–2010) an excess of 4750 suicides occurred in the US, 1000 suicides in England, and 680 suicides in Spain (Corcoran et al, 2015). However, it is not just mental health that is negatively affected by recessions, as many studies worldwide have found that general health indicators also worsen during times of recession (Zavras et al, 2013).

One of the main pathways whereby recessions impact on health is through the adverse relationship between unemployment and health (Bambra, 2011). Unemployment is associated with worse mental health, including suicide (Montgomery et al, 1999a). It has also been linked to higher rates of all-cause mortality as well as limiting long-term illness, and, in some studies, a higher prevalence of risky health behaviours (particularly among young men), including problematic alcohol use and smoking (Montgomery et al, 1999b). Local rates of unemployment are associated with poorer neighbourhood health, and at the country level, increases in the unemployment rate have been associated with increased mortality (Brenner, 1995). Studies from various countries have identified poverty as an important intermediary factor in the relationship between unemployment and health (Bartley et al, 2006). Indeed, the health gap between employed and unemployed people is lower in countries with more generous social security provision (Bambra and Eikemo, 2009).

Some studies of previous economic downturns – including those in the 1970s, 1980s and 1990s as well as the Global Financial Crisis of 2007/8 – suggest that the unemployment – and therefore health – effects of economic downturns can be unequally socially and spatially distributed – thereby exacerbating health inequalities (Bambra et al, 2016). For example, a study in Japan found that economic downturns increased occupational inequalities in general health among men (Kondo et al, 2008). Further, after the Global Financial Crisis, areas of the UK with higher unemployment rates – including the North – had greater increases in suicide rates (Hawton et al, 2016). However, studies have found that recessions do not increase health inequalities in all countries. For example, a Finnish study found that the economic downturn of the 1990s slowed down the trend towards increased socio-economic inequalities in mortality (Valkonen et al, 2000). Similarly, studies of morbidity conducted in Finland, Norway, Sweden, and Denmark found that socio-economic inequalities in general health remained stable in these countries during the 1980s and 1990s – a period marked by economic volatility and recessions (Manderbacka et al, 2001; Dahl and Elstad 2000; Lundberg et al, 2001; Lahlema et al, 2002). Furthermore, a comparative study of trends in general health from 1991–2010 found that there was a more negative impact on the health of those in the lowest educational groups in England – particularly lower educated women – than in Sweden during the recessions of the 1990s and the Global Financial Crisis (Copeland et al, 2013). These findings – of a protective effect of the Scandinavian welfare model – are also supported by a study of inequalities in preterm births in the Scandinavian countries – which remained broadly stable from 1981 to 2000 despite periods of economic downturn (Petersen et al, 2009).

The health inequalities effects of recessions may well therefore be experienced quite differently by otherwise similar people and communities due to national policy variations with more generous welfare systems protecting the health of the population and especially the most vulnerable (Burstrom and Whitehead, 2010). For example, although early analysis of data in South Africa found that the wages of lower educated groups had been impacted by COVID-19 more than the wages of higher educated groups, the financial support provided by the state for poorer households meant that the overall impact on household income in relative terms was less for lower educated households than it was for those with higher levels of education (Channing et al, 2020). Analyses of previous economic downturns suggest that the welfare states in the Social Democratic Scandinavian countries (Denmark, Finland, Norway, Sweden) are particularly good at preventing the deterioration of health of the most vulnerable groups during economic downturns (Bambra, 2011). This may be because the comparatively strong social safety nets they provide buffer against the structural pressures towards widening income and health inequalities (Copeland et al, 2013; Lahlema et al, 2002). The nature of how governments respond – economically and in terms of social and health policy – to the COVID-19 economic crisis (and related crises such as the Cost-of-Living and Energy crisis since 2022) is likely to be very important in terms of the effects it has on regional health inequalities (this is discussed further in Chapter Six).

The economic impacts of COVID-19 can therefore be seen as part of how the pandemic is acting as an unequal syndemic: COVID-19 – as a disease – was exacerbated by existing inequalities, and now – via economic effects – it is in turn creating new inequalities (Bambra et al, 2021a). The unequal economic impacts of the pandemic will have important implications for health inequalities in the medium and longer term – probably more so than the inequalities in COVID-19 itself. However, as the next chapter will explore further, health inequalities can be mitigated by public policy choices.

Conclusion

This chapter has explored the multifaceted potential reasons for why the North was hardest hit by the COVID-19 pandemic. It has argued that the North was left more exposed to the adverse impacts of the pandemic through decades of long-term economic – and health – decline. This meant that the North was least prepared for the pandemic, and it was experienced as a syndemic – whereby COVID-19 exacerbated pre-existing social, economic, and health inequalities. However, the North was more adversely impacted than would be expected based on deprivation alone – with the deep-seated and long-term nature of economic neglect resulting in deprivation amplification. We have also reflected on the role that place (in our case region) plays in shaping intersectional inequalities in health to understand why minority groups and young people in the North fared worse in terms of the parallel pandemic of mental health. Throughout, we have drawn on the health and place literature to examine why the North–South divide pre-pandemic may have exacerbated peri-pandemic inequalities and to reflect on the outcome of the economic impacts on the North on future health inequalities. The next chapter builds on these insights by setting out what can be done to reduce pre-, peri- and post-pandemic regional inequalities in health and what needs to be done to 'Build Back Better'.

SIX

Levelling up and building back better: conclusion

Our book has shown that the COVID-19 pandemic was experienced unequally across the country with the North more exposed and hardest hit – with higher death rates from COVID-19; a more intense experience of the parallel pandemics of mental health, hospital pressure and long COVID; and a worse impact on the economy. The already large regional health and wealth divide in England has been exacerbated by the pandemic. Unless action is taken to rectify this, there is likely to be a long-term health legacy from the COVID-19 crisis – with health inequalities increasing into the future. To avoid a long shadow of COVID-19 hanging over the future of the North, we need to act to reduce the North–South divide. This chapter draws on historical examples of when sizeable reductions in health inequalities have been achieved. Five varied global examples are presented ranging from the 1950s to the 2000s: the Nordic Social Democratic welfare states from the 1950s to 1970s; the Civil Rights Acts and War on Poverty in the 1960s US; democratisation in Brazil in the 1980s; German reunification in the 1990s; and the English Health Inequalities Strategy in the 2000s. From these case studies, three common levelling-up mechanisms whereby health inequalities can be reduced are identified: the expansion of social security and pursuit of a full employment economy; improved access to health care; and enhanced political incorporation.[1] The chapter draws on these to outline what needs to be done now to reduce health inequalities and 'build back better' after the pandemic.

Learning from the past

The first historical example of levelling up health inequalities is the impact of the Social Democratic welfare states in the Nordic countries from the 1950s to the 1970s. After the Second World War, welfare states were established in most European countries, leading to significant improvements to public housing, health care, and the other main social determinants of health including workers enjoying the highest share of national income ever (Eikemo and Bambra, 2008). Post-war welfare states varied and the most encompassing were established in the Nordic countries (Denmark, Finland, Norway, and Sweden) (Bambra, 2011). Their Social Democratic approach was characterised by universal and comparatively generous benefits, collectivism, solidarity (incorporating the working class and the middle classes), a commitment to full employment and income protection, and a strongly interventionist state (Esping-Andersen, 1990). The state was used to promote equality through pre-taxation wage compression organised via strong collective bargaining and the incorporation of the trade union movement within the state; and by using the taxation system to redistribute via the welfare state social security system (Esping-Andersen, 1990). This meant that from the 1950/60s–1980s income inequalities were the smallest – and poverty rates the lowest – this led to lower (absolute) health inequalities in these countries (Ritakallio and Fritzell, 2004). The British Black report of 1980 contained a range of comparative data from the 1970s about health inequalities across Europe. It showed that Norway and Sweden had the smallest (and reducing) socio-economic inequalities in mortality, particularly in comparison to France, West Germany, and the UK (Black et al, 1980). Other comparative studies of mortality conducted in the 1970s and 1980s came to similar conclusions. For example, a study of educational inequalities in mortality in six European countries in the 1970s found that relative inequalities were largest in France, then the UK and Finland while they were smallest in Denmark, Norway and Sweden (Valkonen, 1989). This was reinforced by subsequent studies of morbidity which compared Sweden and the UK (Lundberg, 1986; Vagero and Lundberg, 1989). In this period, the Nordic countries also had the lowest mortality rates across all social classes (Lundberg and Lahelma, 2001). However, this 'golden age' of the welfare state effectively ended with the economic crisis of the 1970s and the emergence of neoliberal economics – initially in the Anglo-American countries but then spreading across continental Europe in the 1980s and 1990s (as noted in Chapter One). Neoliberalism led to the erosion of the post-war Social Democratic welfare model and an increase in income (and health) inequalities (Schrecker and Bambra, 2015).

The second example comes from the US in the 1960s when President Lyndon B. Johnson announced the 'Great Society' policy programme which led to a series of substantial programmes to address inequalities in health care, civil rights, education, and poverty (Andrew, 1998). The Medicare (1965 – universal health insurance for all over 65s) and Medicaid (1966 – limited health care costs coverage for welfare recipients) programmes were introduced (Holt, 1999). These substantially increased access to health care for the poorest groups (Holt, 1999). The 'War on Poverty' included various initiatives to address urban and rural poverty; increased educational opportunities (including significant increases in Federal funding for the education system); expanded the Federal food stamp programme;

increased the value of the state pension; and expanded the scope of the main Federal welfare programme – Aid for Dependent Children – to cover African American mothers (Karger and Stoesz, 1990). The 1964 Civil Rights Acts outlawed racial discrimination (which led to the abolition of the legal system of racial discrimination in the 21 Southern States and District of Columbia called 'Jim Crow') leading to the desegregation of schools and public accommodations (including hospitals), equalised voting rights and led to increased wages in the South (Packard, 2003; Beardsley, 1986). A series of analyses by Krieger and colleagues (2008, 2014, 2017) has examined the impact of these reforms on health inequalities. They found that racial and income inequalities in premature mortality (deaths under age 75) and infant mortality rates (IMR)[2] declined between 1966 and 1980 after the 'War on Poverty' and the enactment of civil rights legislation. The positive impact of Jim Crow abolition has also been demonstrated with regards to racial inequalities in cancer rates (Krieger et al, 2017). Health inequalities in the US then increased again between 1980 and 2002 during the Reagan-Bush period of neoliberalism when public welfare services (including health care insurance coverage) were cut, funding of social assistance was reduced, the minimum wage was frozen and the tax base was shifted from the rich to the poor leading to increased income inequalities (see Chapter One) (Schrecker and Bambra, 2015).

The process of democratisation and welfare expansion in Brazil from the 1980s to the 2000s provides our third example. In 1985, Brazil started a gradual transition from military dictatorship (1964–1985) to become a stable democracy by the mid-2000s. This increased political participation was accompanied by an expansion of health and welfare programmes, including the introduction of universal health care in 1988 (the Unified Health System); a National Women's Health Programme and National Programme for Child Health in 1984; a Family Health

Program in 1994; a National Programme for the Reduction of Infant Mortality in 1995; and the Bolsa Família cash transfer programme for low-income women with children in 2003. These led to a significant improvement in maternal and child health care and a reduction in Brazil's poverty rates as well as a decrease in income inequalities between rich and poor (Macinko et al, 2006; Landmann Szwarcwald et al, 2020; Victora et al, 2011). Since these reforms, IMR in Brazil fell by more than 70 per cent between 1980 and 2015 (Landmann Szwarcwald et al, 2020). This is one of the fastest drops in infant mortality ever recorded worldwide and higher than would be expected by the increase in Brazil's GDP per capita (Victora et al, 2011). Regional differences in IMR and differences between rich and poor social groups also decreased (Landmann Szwarcwald et al, 2020). For example, the gap in IMR between the top and bottom wealth quintiles more than halved between 1991 and 2002 (Victora et al, 2011). Other indicators of child health inequalities – such as stunted growth – also improved significantly during this period (Monteiro et al, 2009). However, Brazil's reductions in health inequalities and improvements in population health are under threat from the economic and political crises in the country since 2015. Brazil experienced a significant economic recession in 2015 which was followed by the implementation of austerity measures including a substantial reduction in expenditure on – and population coverage of – social welfare programmes – including Bolsa Família, leading to an increase in poverty rates. Democracy has also declined in Brazil since the election of President Jair Bolsonaro in the 2018 election and the country also suffered significantly during the COVID-19 pandemic.

The fall of Communism and the reunification of Germany in the 1990s provides a further example of how to reduce regional health inequalities – significantly, at scale and in a fairly short time frame. In 1990, the life expectancy gap between the former East and the former West of Germany was almost three years for women and three and a half years for men. This gap rapidly narrowed in the following decades so that by 2010 it had dwindled to just a few months for women and just over one year for men (Bambra, 2016). This was achieved through a variety of mechanisms. First, living standards of East Germans improved with increases in wage levels and better access to a variety of foods and consumer goods (Gjonça et al, 2000). This particularly benefitted old age pensioners in the East as the West German pension system was extended into the East which resulted in huge increases in income for older East Germans (Nolte et al, 2002). Research by the Max Planck Institute for Demographic Research in Rostock has shown that the rapid improvement in life expectancy in 1990s East Germany was largely a result of falling death rates among pensioners (Nolte et al, 2002). Second, immediately after reunification, considerable financial support was given to modernise the hospitals and health care equipment in the East and the availability of nursing care, screening, and pharmaceuticals also increased. This raised standards of health care in the East so that they were comparable to those of the West within just a few years (Nolte et al, 2002). This had notable impacts on, for example, improvements in neonatal mortality in East and in mortality from conditions amenable to prevention (for example cancer screening) or medical treatment (Nolte et al, 2000). Both the improvement in living standards and the increased investment in health care were the result of the deep and sustained *political* decision to reunify Germany as fully as possible so that – in the words of the German Chancellor Helmut Kohl (1982–1998) – "what belongs together will grow together" (Bambra, 2016). Indeed, the improvements in the East were funded by a special Solidarity Surcharge – an additional income tax charge paid across Germany (Bambra, 2016).

Our final case study is the most recent – England's National Health Inequalities Strategy in the 2000s. In 1997, a Labour government (Social Democratic) was elected in the UK on a manifesto that included a commitment to reducing health inequalities. This led to the implementation – between 2000 and 2010 – of a wide-ranging and multifaceted health inequalities reduction strategy for England in which policymakers systematically and explicitly attempted to reduce inequalities in health. The strategy focused specifically on: supporting families, engaging communities in tackling deprivation, improving prevention, increasing access to health care, and reducing child and pensioner poverty rates as well as tackling the underlying social determinants of health (Holdroyd et al, 2022). For example, the strategy included large increases in levels of public spending on a range of social programmes, the introduction of the national minimum wage, a child poverty strategy, an increase in pension rates, area-based interventions such as the Health Action Zones, and a substantial increase in expenditure on the health care system (Whitehead and Popay, 2010). These policies led to reductions in social inequalities in the key social determinants of health – including unemployment, child poverty, housing quality, access to health care, and educational attainment (Bambra, 2016). These were accompanied by modest reductions in health inequalities between the most deprived areas in England and the rest of the country: inequalities in life expectancy decreased by just over a year for men and around six months for women (Barr et al, 2017); the gap in IMR narrowed by 12 deaths per 100,000 births per year (Robinson et al, 2019); and inequalities in mortality amendable to health care interventions decreased by 35 deaths per 100,000 for men and 16 deaths per 100,000 for women (Barr et al, 2014). The strategy may have been even more effective if it had been sustained over a longer time period – but from 2010 the newly elected Conservative-Liberal coalition government pursued a policy of austerity which has been associated with increasing poverty, income inequality, and health inequalities (Taylor-Robinson et al, 2019).

The three levellers of health inequalities

Reading across these five varied case studies, it is possible to identify three common 'levellers': welfare state expansion, improved health care access, and enhanced political incorporation. Common to all five examples is the expansion of social security safety nets (and the reduction of poverty) and increased health care access particularly for the poorest groups. Likewise, four of our examples (Nordic countries, the US, Brazil, and Germany) are characterised by the political incorporation of the working classes and/or minority groups. Further evidence of the importance of these three mechanisms for reducing health inequalities comes from studies of the health effects of the opposite – when reductions in social security and health care provision have been associated with increases in health inequalities. For example, Krieger's analysis of time trends in inequalities in IMR and premature mortality in the US found that while inequalities decreased during a period of welfare state enhancements, they increased again when social security was reduced in the 1980s (Krieger et al, 2008). Similar associations have been found between the expansion and contraction of the welfare state and post-war trends in health inequalities in the UK and New Zealand (Scott-Samuel et al, 2014; Shaw et al, 2005). More recent research into the impact of austerity policies in Europe has also found that health inequalities increased (Niedzwiedz et al, 2016; Akhter et al, 2018). For example, as child poverty decreased between 2000 and 2010 in England, inequalities in IMR decreased (Robinson et al, 2019). However, as child poverty rates increased between 2010 and 2020 – the decade of austerity – inequalities in IMR increased again (Taylor-Robinson et al, 2019). This 'dose–response' relationship between social security provision and health inequalities has been confirmed by a large international systematic review (Simpson et al, 2021). So, there is an association between the 'waxing and waning' of the welfare state and health inequalities: as welfare state provision increases (and poverty decreases), health inequalities fall; when the welfare state is reduced (and poverty rates increase), health inequalities tend to increase.

These three mechanisms are not independent of one another though – historically, democratisation and the political incorporation of the working classes and minority groups has tended to result in increases in welfare state and health care provision (Beckfield, 2018). The case studies have also highlighted the need for policy action to be sustained over long periods of time (the five examples all span at least a decade) and for there to be sufficient political will to sustain it.

These examples could therefore help us to develop more effective post-pandemic public health policy programmes.

Recommendations: A new national health inequalities strategy

Drawing on these historical examples and the results of our analyses, here we make a specific recommendation for how to 'build back better' to reduce regional health inequalities: a new national health inequalities strategy is urgently needed to reduce the regional health and wealth divide and prevent health inequalities growing post-pandemic.

The COVID-19 pandemic hit the North of England hardest: people in the region were more likely to die from the virus than those elsewhere and they suffered more from the 'collateral damage' of mental health, hospital disruption, long COVID and economic upheaval. Pre-existing economic and health inequalities account for many of the reasons for why the North suffered the most and the impact of the pandemic means that the situation is getting worse. Post-pandemic, the North is less resilient than it was pre-pandemic, and it was already in a disadvantaged state of health and wealth. Emerging from the pandemic, the UK is in a pivotal position where it can use the learnings of the past to build a stronger, healthier society across the whole of the country – or not. Post-pandemic we are facing new threats to health and wealth – an unprecedented NHS waiting list (with over 6.7 million patients waiting for operations at the time of writing in July 2022) and ever reducing day-to-day access; the cost of living crisis (with high inflation impacting on the household budgets of increasing numbers of people); climate change (with heat waves and potential food shortages); the Russian war on Ukraine (fuelling inflation and food shortages) as well as longer term threats to health security such as the spread of infectious diseases (for example the Monkey Pox epidemic in 2022) and the background threat of anti-microbial resistance. Against this extreme back drop, the country needs to unite again – and show the spirit of solidarity we generated during the COVID-19 lockdowns – to protect the more vulnerable people, communities, and regions. But we are also in danger of ignoring the factors which have led to the devastating impact of COVID-19 in the North of England and allowing these future threats to leave it even further behind.

To address this, a national health inequalities strategy is needed again. It should focus on tackling the key social determinants of health inequalities across the life course and across the country – as well as increasing NHS provision – particularly in the North. Drawing on the evidence of the past – and considering future challenges – the strategy should include the following recommendations:

Social policy recommendations:

- A commitment to ending child poverty – key early interventions could include increasing the value of welfare payments for families with children; extending the provision of free childcare; extending the provision of free school meals; and investing in children's services by increasing government grants to the most deprived local authorities, particularly those in the North.
- Reduce poverty rates across the population by increasing the value of out-of-work social security benefits (for example

Universal Credit); providing support for household fuel costs to combat the cost-of-living crisis; increasing the national minimum wage; and ensuring that the state pension prevents old age poverty.

- Introduce a publicly funded social care service to support families and reduce pressure on the NHS.

Health care policy recommendations:

- Invest in increasing capacity in Northern hospitals to help them catch-up on non-COVID-19 health care and reduce the historically unprecedented NHS waiting list.
- Provide additional resource to local authorities and the NHS in deprived areas (especially those in the North), by increasing the health inequalities weighting within the NHS funding formula.
- Deliver a ring-fenced budget to tackle health inequalities at a regional level and increase local authority public health funding to address the higher levels of deprivation and public health need in the North. This could include creating Northern 'Health for Life' centres offering a life-long programme of health and wellbeing advice and support services from pre-natal to healthy ageing programmes.

Mental health policy recommendations:

- Increase NHS and local authority resources and service provision for addressing mental health in the North – with additional, tailored, outreach services for young people and people from ethnic minority communities in the North.
- Integrated Care Systems should commission more health promotion, condition management, and prevention services that promote the health and wellbeing of people in the North.
- Invest in research into the impacts of mental health interventions in the North, specifically in communities which will benefit most strongly from them.

Public health policy recommendations:

- Develop a place-based pandemic preparedness plan which safeguards vulnerable groups such as those in care homes, with disabilities and those with chronic ill health and living in regions with the highest need.
- NHS England and the Office for Health improvement and Disparities should adopt a public mental health approach that focuses on early mental ill health prevention.
- Restore local authority public health budgets to pre-austerity levels with particular boosts in funding into more deprived areas in the North.

Political and economic policy recommendations:

- Increase the devolution of political power to local communities to increase community voice, influence and address the democratic deficit in the regions.
- Implement a 'green new deal' industrial strategy – to increase our resilience to climate change while also increasing employment, with investment targeted into job creation in the North.
- Health needs to be put at the heart of *all* policy making and Health Equity Impact Assessments should be embedded in all policy processes to ensure that future investments do not exacerbate regional inequalities.

Only a radical, extensive, and long-term national health inequalities strategy such as this can do what needs to be done to build a stronger, healthier, more equal country and a North that is more resilient to the future threats to health and wealth.

Notes

one

[1] For a wider discussion of how to define the North, see Bambra (2016).

[2] This is apparent in the literary works of the times particularly those of Charles Dickens (for example, *Hard Times*, 1854 or *A Tale of Two Cities*, 1859) and Elizabeth Gaskell (for example, *North and South*, 1855).

[3] Socio-economic status is a term that refers to occupational class, income, or educational level (Bambra, 2011).

[4] The materialist explanation focuses on income and on what income enables – access to goods and services and exposures to material (physical) risk factors (for example, poor housing, inadequate diet, physical hazards at work, environmental exposures). Psychosocial explanations focus on how social inequality makes people feel – domination/subordination, superiority/ inferiority, social support, demands and control – and the effects of the biological consequences of these feelings on health. The behavioural explanation considers the association between socio-economic status and health to be a result of health-related behaviours because of adverse personal/psychological characteristics or because unhealthy behaviours may be more culturally acceptable among lower socio-economic groups (Bartley, 2016; Skalická et al, 2009).

[5] For a more detailed overview of the history of the North South divide, see Bambra (2016).

[6] Keynesian economic ideology is characterised by full employment, public ownership of industry, and an active role for the state in social policy (for example, a universal welfare state). For more detail, see Schrecker and Bambra (2015).

[7] Neoliberalism was also pursued in the US in the 1980s by President Ronald Reagan and Chancellor Helmut Kohl in West Germany.

[8] Deindustrialisation was implemented as a 'shock doctrine' in the UK with very rapid loss of employment within a few years. In other Western European countries, it was phased in more gradually and often with more

safety nets (such as employment services or inducements for new industry to come to the affected areas) (Bambra, 2016).

[9] For example, the value of unemployment benefits fell from 54 per cent of average wages in 1971 to 20 per cent or less in every year post-1990 (Scruggs et al, 2014).

[10] A more detailed overview of neoliberalism and its health impacts is provided by Schrecker and Bambra (2015).

[11] The financial crisis of 2007/8 was the worst economic period for 60 years (Gamble, 2009).

[12] UK wealth has increasingly been concentrated among the top 0.1 per cent (one one-thousandth) of the population – their share of wealth has increased from seven per cent in 1978 to over 25 per cent today (Saez and Zucman, 2014).

[13] For example, Blackpool, in the North West of England, was hit worst of all – with an estimated loss of more than £900 a year for every adult of working age in the town (Beatty and Fothergill, 2014).

[14] The North West voted 53.7 per cent Yorkshire and The Humber 57.7 per cent and the North East 58 per cent compared to a national average of 52 per cent. www.bbc.co.uk/news/uk-politics-36616028

[15] Lower super output areas are small geographical units used in official government statistics. They have been artificially generated to be consistent in population size – the minimum population is 1000 and the mean is 1500.

[16] The Index of Multiple Deprivation is the most common measure of area-level deprivation. It produces a ranking of areas in England based on relative local scores for: income, employment, health, education, crime, access to services and living environment.

[17] The Northern Health Science Alliance is a health and life sciences partnership between the leading NHS trusts, universities, and Academic Health Science Networks in northern England.

two

[1] Births, deaths, and marriages dataset: COVID-19 deaths by local area and deprivation. www.ons.gov.uk/peoplepopulationandcommunity/births deathsandmarriages/deaths/datasets/deathsduetocovid19bylocalarea anddeprivation

[2] We use the latest available data reflecting the 13-month period (March 2020 to March 2021). We stop at March 2021 as mortality rates attributable to COVID-19 become small from April 2021.

[3] The ONS use ICD10 codes 'U07.1' and 'U07.2' to define deaths where COVID-19 was the underlying cause. These deaths due to COVID-19 only include deaths where COVID-19 was the underlying (main) cause.

Deaths 'due to other causes' includes any deaths where the underlying cause was not COVID-19; this category may include some deaths where the underlying cause was not COVID-19 but COVID-19 was mentioned on the death certificate as a contributory cause of death.

[4] The 'Age structure' and 'Ethnic structure' of each LAD was determined by a series of variables indicating what percentage of the local authority's population were in pre-defined age groups and ethic groups. These data were taken from the 2011 Census to avoid issues associated with extrapolating to non-Census years. We have repeated our analysis using the estimated values for 2019, and the results are qualitatively very similar. Age-standardised mortality rates were not provided at MSOA level and so we constructed the mortality rate per 10,000 population by dividing the total count of deaths attributable to COVID-19 by the 2019 population estimate and multiplying by 10,000.

[5] By definition, this group of people were thought of as being 'high-risk' and so we use this as a proxy for underlying health status. Areas with higher rates of people shielding will, by definition, have higher levels of ill-health than areas with lower rates of people shielding. We have used other measures of population health and the results are qualitatively very similar.

[6] https://digital.nhs.uk/data-and-information/publications/statistical/mi-engl ish-coronavirus-covid-19-shielded-patient-list-summary-totals

[7] Specifically, we estimate four regression models:

Model 1: $Outcome_l = \beta(The\ North_l) + \varepsilon_l$

Model 2: $Outcome_l = \beta(The\ North_l) + \gamma(Age\ structure_l) + \varepsilon_l$

Model 3: $Outcome_l = \beta(The\ North_l) + \gamma(Age\ structure_l) + \lambda(Ethnic\ structure_l) + \varepsilon_l$

Model 4: $Outcome_l = \beta(The\ North_l) + \gamma(Age\ structure_l) + \lambda(Ethnic\ structure_l) + \delta(IMD\ quintile_l) + \mu(Patient\ shielding\ rate_l) + \varepsilon_l$

where subscript I refers to each unique LAD, Outcome is the COVID-19 mortality rate, 'The North' is a binary variable that takes the value 1 if a LAD is in the North region and 0 otherwise (that is, if a local authority is in the rest of England), 'Age structure' is a series of variables indicating what percentage of the local authority's population is in pre-defined age-groups, 'Ethnic structure' is a series of variables indicating what percentage of the local authority's population belong to pre-defined ethic-groups, 'IMD quintile' is a categorical variable indicating the relative deprivation of the LAD, and 'Patient shielding rate' is a variable indicating the rate of patient shielding per 10,000 in the local authority. This can be thought of as a measure of the underlying health status of the population.

[8] The full results are contained in table A1.3 in in our report here: (Munford et al, 2021). www.thenhsa.co.uk/app/uploads/2021/09/A-Year-of-COVID-in-the-North-report-2021.pdf (Munford et al, 2021).

[9] $100 \times (29.4 - 15.2) / 15.2 = 48.299\%$.

[10] High is defined as above the mean and low is defined as below the mean.

[11] Middle super output areas (MSOAs) are small geographical units used in official government statistics. They have been artificially generated to be consistent in population size – the minimum population is 5000 and the mean is 7200. We used MSOAs because this is the smallest geographical scale at which COVID-19 death data is publicly available.

three

[1] We acknowledge that anti-depressant prescribing rates are not necessarily the ideal indicator of depression prevalence as they may be used for a diverse range of illnesses (including panic disorder, stress incontinence, menopausal symptoms, or neuropathic pain). Therefore, we acknowledge that relying on the prescription of these medications may overestimate the likely prevalence of depression. However, we have no reason to assume that this would affect the North and the rest of England in a differential way, and hence don't think it should in any way bias our results or interpretation.

[2] Understanding Society: Waves 1–10, 2009–2019 and Harmonised BHPS: Waves 1–18, 1991–2009, 13th Edition. Data collection, University of Essex, 2021. Institute for Social and Economic Research, N.S.R., Kantar Public.

[3] The UKHLS has a complex and multi-stage sampling frame and includes a boost sample to increase the sample size of participants from an ethnic minority background. Further detail on the sample design of the survey is available online. www.iser.essex.ac.uk/research/publications/working-papers/understanding-society/2009-01

[4] These covered April to July 2020, September 2020, November 2020, January 2021, March 2021 and September 2021.

[5] The 'caseness' measure recodes 1 and 2 values to zero and 3 and 4 values to 1, so that when summed the scale runs from 1 to 12.

[6] 'Caseness' measures are relevant to clinical mental health contexts. For example, the 'Improving Access to Psychological Therapies' service in the NHS delivers psychological therapies for people with common mental health disorders (CMDs). On accepting referrals, self-reported mental health questionnaires for CMDs such as anxiety and depression are used. Individuals who score above the clinical cut-off are then classed as a clinical case (https://fingertips.phe.org.uk/profile/common-mental-disorders/supporting-information/Glossary).

NOTES

[7] Net household income was adjusted for household size and composition by following as closely as possible the practice used in the OECD equivalence scale used in the main UKHLS data set: a weight of 1 was assigned to the first adult in every household, 0.5 to all subsequent adults and 0.3 to each person aged 15 or under. Net household income was then divided by the household sum of this weight.

[8] The language used in the reporting of these analyses to refer to people from ethnic minority backgrounds was chosen to most accurately reflect the analytical operationalisation of ethnicity used in the quantitative analyses performed. Descriptive analyses showed the sample sizes of any smaller aggregations of the ethnicity categories available in the dataset to be too small to provide reliable results. Tables presenting sample size statistics by region and ethnicity are included in the appendix (tables 6.1 and 6.2) of our full report (Bambra et al, 2022). The authors acknowledge the limitations of this approach and understand that those described by the term 'ethnic minority' in this book are not a homogenous group. A greater volume of data and further research is required to understand the nuances of the impact of COVID-19 on the mental health of more fine-grained and meaningful ethnic groupings.

[9] The full descriptive statistics are available in table 2.1 in our report here: www.thenhsa.co.uk/app/uploads/2022/07/NHSA-MENTAL-HEALTH-REPORT.pdf

[10] This includes: tricyclic and related anti-depressant drugs, monoamineoxidase inhibitors, selective serotonin re-uptake inhibitors, and other anti-depressant drugs. For more details, see https://opendata.nhsbsa.net/dataset/english-prescribing-data-epd

[11] CCGs are clinically-led statutory NHS bodies that have a responsibility for the planning and commissioning of health care services in their local area. They were created following the Health and Social Care Act in 2012, and replaced Primary Care Trusts on 1 April 2013. The number of CCGs has fluctuated over time following mergers. In the dataset we use, there are 106 CCGs in England.

[12] Each CCG is located entirely within an NHS region. There are seven NHS regions, which differ slightly from the nine government office regions: East of England, London, Midlands, North East and Yorkshire, North West, South East and South West.

[13] A difference-in-difference model is a form of a 'controlled before-and-after' design.

[14] Difference-in-difference involves estimating models of the form:

$$y_{it}=\alpha+\beta North_i+\gamma After_t+\delta(North*After)_{it}+\pi_t+\varepsilon_{it}$$

where y_{it} is the per-person prescription of anti-depressant medication in CCG i in month t, $North_i$ is a binary variable equal to one if CCG i is in the North of England and zero for the rest of England, $After_t$ is a binary variable equal to one if the month of observation is during the pandemic (March 2020 or later) and zero for pre-pandemic months. The interaction term is equal to one if and only if the observation relates to a Northern CCG in a pandemic month. The key parameter of interest is δ and it tells us if there were differential effects of the pandemic experienced between the North and the rest of England. We additionally included year and month-fixed effects to account for seasonal variation.

[15] Difference in difference estimation of the effect of the pandemic on the prescription of ant-depressants: Coefficient (and 95% CI) North 1.05 (0.99 to 1.10, p<0.001), After 0.13 (−0.18 to 0.29), North*After 0.12 (0.03 to 0.21, p<0.1), N=120. The model is estimated using OLS with robust standard errors, clustered at the level of aggregation (North/rest of England). The same size indicates there are 120 monthly observations observed in two groups (North and rest of England). The model also includes fixed effects for years and months.

[16] Available here: www.england.nhs.uk/statistics/statistical-work-areas/covid-19-hospital-activity/

[17] Our models were informed by a conceptual framework. In the conceptual framework, the key exposure is 'live in the North' and the key outcomes are those related to COVID-19. To obtain estimates for the outlined conceptual framework, we run four models: Model 1: $Outcome_i = \beta(The\ North_i) + \varepsilon_i$; Model 2: $Outcome_i = \beta(The\ North_i) + \gamma(Age\ structure_i) + \varepsilon_i$; Model 3: $Outcome_i = \beta(The\ North_i) + \gamma(Age\ structure_i) + \lambda(Ethnic\ structure_i) + \varepsilon_i$; Model 4: $Outcome_i = \beta(The\ North_i) + \gamma(Age\ structure_i) + \lambda(Ethnic\ structure_i) + \delta(IMD\ quintile_i) + \mu(Patient\ shielding\ rate) + \varepsilon_i$. Where: Subscript I refers to each unique local authority district; 'Outcome' is the proportion of hospital beds occupied by COVID-19 patients during the pandemic (April 2020 to March 2021); 'The North' is a binary variable that takes the value 1 if a local authority is in the North region and 0 otherwise; 'Age structure' is a series of variables from the Census indicating what percentage of the local authority's population is in pre-defined age-groups; 'Ethnic structure' is a series of variables indicating what percentage of the local authority's population belong to pre-defined ethic-groups; 'IMD quintile' is a categorical variable indicating the relative deprivation of the local authority; 'Patient shielding rate' is variables indicating the rate of patient shielding per 10,000 in the local authority. This can be thought of as a measure of the underlying health status of the population.

[18] To ease interpretation, we present the results of the statistical models as graphics in proportions and state the coefficients as percentage point increases.

[19] Available at: www.ons.gov.uk/peoplepopulationandcommunity/healthan dsocialcare/conditionsanddiseases/datasets/alldatarelatingtoprevalenceo fongoingsymptomsfollowingcoronaviruscovid19infectionintheuk

[20] These survey estimates relate to self-reported long COVID, as experienced by study participants, rather than clinically diagnosed ongoing symptomatic COVID-19 or post-COVID-19 syndrome. Study participants were asked to respond to the following questions: 'Would you describe yourself as having "long COVID", that is, you are still experiencing symptoms more than 4 weeks after you first had COVID-19, that are not explained by something else?' and, if so: 'Does this reduce your ability to carry-out day-to-day activities compared with the time before you had COVID-19?' and 'Have you had any of the following symptoms as part of your experience of long COVID? Please include any pre-existing symptoms which long COVID has made worse' (ONS, 2022).

four

[1] From: www.ons.gov.uk/employmentandlabourmarket/peoplenotinwork/ unemployment/datasets/claimantcountbyunitaryandlocalauthorityexper imental/current

[2] 80 per cent of wages up to a cap of £2,500 per month with employers expected to make up the additional 20 per cent.

[3] www.gov.uk/government/statistics/coronavirus-job-retention-scheme-sta tistics-3-june-2021

[4] A time trend of the uptake of furlough is shown in Munford et al, 2021.

[5] www.nomisweb.co.uk/. Original data are from the Annual Study of Hours and Earnings (ASHE).

[6] We additionally exclude London as it is well known that wages are much higher there, due to the service and financial nature of many of the employers located there.

[7] See Bambra et al, 2018, p 27, figure 5.2.

[8] https://pldr.org/dataset/2noyv/small-area-mental-health-index-samhi

[9] GVA is a local version of GDP. Here, GVA was deflated to 2018 prices to remove any possible inflationary changes.

[10] The use of fixed-effects models allowed us to isolate the within-area changes in mental well-being and how they correlated with the within-area changes in GVA. This allowed us to abstract away from factors that were largely time-invariant (that is, deprivation and need).

[11] 95% CI: £685.37 to £2,298.31.

five

[1] This section is based on Bambra et al (2021b), reproduced under Commons Creative Licence.

2 These consequences of socio-economic inequality also intersect with ethnicity, as ethnic minorities are much more likely to be socio-economically deprived and/or to live in more deprived neighbourhoods, as well as to be disproportionally disadvantaged by compounding determinants (Bambra et al, 2021b).

3 By way of example, a recent systematic review of intersectional inequalities in mental health found only 20 studies and that 'few studies analysed factors potentially explaining the intersectional inequalities' (Fagrell Trygg, Gustafsson and Månsdotter, 2019).

six

1 This section is based on Bambra (2021) Levelling up: Global examples of reducing health inequalities. *Scandinavian Journal of Public Health.* doi:10.1177/14034948211022428, under the terms of the Creative Commons Attribution 4.0 License.

2 Infant mortality rates (IMR) are defined as deaths before age one.

References

Adams, O. (1981) *Health and Economic Activity: A Time-Series Analysis of Canadian Mortality and Unemployment Rates*, Ottawa: Health Division, Statistics Canada.

Akhter, N., Bambra, C., Mattheys, K., Warren, J. and Kasim, A. (2018) Inequalities in mental health and well-being in a time of austerity: Longitudinal findings from the Stockton-on-Tees cohort study, *SSM Pop Health*, 6: 75–84.

Albani, V., Welsh, C., Brown, H., Matthews, F., and Bambra, C. (2022) Explaining the deprivation gap in COVID-19 mortality rates: A decomposition analysis of geographical inequalities, *England, Social Science & Medicine*, 115319.

Almeida, M., Shrestha, A.D., Stojanac, D., and Miller, L.J. (2020) The impact of the COVID-19 pandemic on women's mental health, *Archives of Women's Mental Health*, 23(6): 741–748.

Alqahtani, J., Oyelade, T., Aldhahir, A., Alghamdi, S., Almehmadi, M., Alqahtani, A., Quaderi, S., Mandal, S., Hurst, J. (2020) Prevalence, severity and mortality associated with COPD and smoking in patients with COVID-19: a rapid systematic review and meta-analysis, *PLoS ONE*, 15(5): e0233147.

Andrew, J. (1998) *Lyndon Johnson and the Great Society*, Chicago: Ivan R Dee.

Baker, A. and Billinge, M. (2004) *Geographies of England: The North-South Divide, Imagined and Material*, Cambridge, Cambridge University Press.

Bambra, C. (2011) *Work, Worklessness, and the Political Economy of Health*, Oxford: Oxford University Press.

Bambra, C. (2016) *Health Divides: Where You Live Can Kill You*, Bristol: Policy Press.

Bambra, C. (2022a) Placing intersectional inequalities in health, *Health and Place*, 75: 102761.

Bambra, C. (2022b) Pandemic inequalities: Emerging infectious diseases and health equity, *International Journal of Equity in Health*, 21: 6.

Bambra, C. and Eikemo, T. (2009) Welfare state regimes, unemployment and health: A comparative study of the relationship between unemployment and self-reported health in 23 European countries, *Journal of Epidemiology and Community Health*, 63: 92–98.

Bambra, C. and Orton, C. (2016) A train journey through the English health divide: topological map, *Environment and Planning A*, 48: 811–814.

Bambra, C., Fox, D., and Scott-Samuel, A. (2005) Towards a politics of health, *Health Promotion International*, 20: 187–193.

Bambra, C., Barr, B., and Milne, E. (2014a) North and South: Addressing the English health divide, *Journal of Public Health*, 36: 183–186.

Bambra, C., Robertson, S., Kasim, A., Smith, J., Cairns-Nagi, J., Copeland, A., Finlay, N., and Johnson., K. (2014b) Healthy land? An examination of the area-level association between brownfield land and morbidity and mortality in England, *Environment and Planning A*, 46: 433–454.

Bambra, C., Garthwaite, K., Copeland, A., and Barr, B. (2016) All in it together? Health Inequalities, Welfare Austerity and the 'Great Recession', in K.E. Smith, S. Hill, and C. Bambra (eds) *Health Inequalities: Critical Perspectives*, Oxford: Oxford University Press, pp 164–176.

Bambra, C., Munford, L., Brown, H., Wilding, A., Robinson, T., Holland, P., Barr, B., Hill, H., Regan, M., Rice, N., and Sutton, M. (2018) *Health for Wealth: Building a Healthier Northern Powerhouse for UK Productivity*, Newcastle: Northern Health Sciences Alliance. www.thenhsa.co.uk/app/uploads/2018/11/NHSA-REPORT-FINAL.pdf [accessed 08/08/22].

Bambra, C., Smith, K., and Pearce, J. (2019) Scaling up: The politics of health and place, *Social Science & Medicine*, 232: 36–42.

Bambra, C., Riordan, R., Ford, J., and Matthews, F. (2020a) The COVID-19 pandemic and health inequalities, *Journal of Epidemiology and Community Health*, 74: 964–968.

Bambra, C., Munford, L., Alexandros, A., Barr, B., Brown, H., Davies, H., Konstantinos, D., Mason, K., Pickett, K., Taylor, C., Taylor-Robinson, D., and Wickham, S. (2020b) *COVID-19 and the Northern Powerhouse: Tackling Inequalities for UK Health and Productivity*, Newcastle: NHSA. www.thenhsa.co.uk/app/uplo ads/2020/11/NP-COVID-REPORT-101120-.pdf [accessed 08/08/22].

Bambra, C., Smith, K., and Lynch, J. (2021a) *The Unequal Pandemic: COVID-19 and Health Inequalities*, Bristol: Policy Press.

Bambra, C., Albani, V., and Franklin, P. (2021b) COVID-19 and the gender health paradox, *Scandinavian Journal of Public Health*, 49: 17–26.

Bambra, C., Munford, L., Bennett, N., Khavandi, S., Davies, H., Bernard, K., Akhter, N., Pickett, K., and Taylor-Robinson, D. (2022) *The Parallel Pandemic: COVID-19 and Mental Health, Project Report*, Newcastle: Northern Health Science Alliance. www.then hsa.co.uk/app/uploads/2022/07/NHSA-MENTAL-HEALTH-REPORT.pdf [accessed 08/08/22].

Barnes, M.C., Donovan, J.L., Wilson, C., Chatwin, J., Davies, R., Potokar, J. et al (2017) Seeking help in times of economic hardship: Access, experiences of services and unmet need, *BMC Psychiatry*, 17: 84.

Barr, B., Taylor-Robinson, D., Scott-Samuel, A., McKee, M., and Stuckler, D. (2012) Suicides associated with the 2008–10 economic recession in England: time trend analysis, *British Medical Journal*, 345(7873): e5142.

Barr, B., Bambra, C., and Whitehead M. (2014) The impact of NHS resource allocation policy on health inequalities in England 2001–11: Longitudinal ecological study, *British Medical Journal*, 348(7960): g3231.

Barr, B., Higgerson, J., and Whitehead, M. (2017) Investigating the impact of the English health inequalities strategy: Time trend analysis, *British Medical Journal*, 8116(358): j3310.

Bartley, M. (2016) *Health Inequality: An Introduction to Concepts, Theories and Methods*, Cambridge: Polity Press.

Bartley, M., Ferrie, J. and Montgomery, S.M. (2006) Health and labour market disadvantage: Unemployment, non-employment, and job insecurity, in M. Marmot and R.G. Wilkinson (eds) *Social Determinants of Health*, Oxford: Oxford University Press, pp 78–96.

Bauer, G. (2014) Incorporating intersectionality theory into population health research methodology: Challenges and the potential to advance health equity, *Social Science & Medicine*, 110: 10–17.

Bauer, G. and Scheima, A. (2019) The Intersectional Discrimination Index: Development and validation of measures of self-reported enacted and anticipated discrimination for intercategorical analysis, *Social Science & Medicine*, 226: 225–235.

Bauer, G., Churchill, S.M., Mahendran, M., Walwyn, C., Lizotte, D., and Villa-Rueda, A.A. (2021) Intersectionality in quantitative research: A systematic review of its emergence and applications of theory and methods, *SSM-Population Health*, 14: 100798.

Beardsley, E.H. (1986) Good-bye to Jim Crow: The desegregation of Southern hospitals, 1945–70, *Bull Hist Med.*, 60: 367–386.

Beatty, C. and Fothergill, S. (2014) The local and regional impact of the UK's welfare reforms, *Cambridge Journal of Regions Economy and Society*, 7: 63–79.

Bécares, L. and Nazroo, J. (2013) Social capital, ethnic density and mental health among ethnic minority people in England: A mixed-methods study, *Ethnicity & Health*, 18(6): 544–562.

Bécares, L., Cormack, D., and Harris, R. (2013) Ethnic density and area deprivation: Neighbourhood effects on Māori health and racial discrimination in Aotearoa/New Zealand, *Social Science & Medicine*, 88: 76–82.

Beckfield, J. (2018) *Political Sociology and the People's Health*, New York: Oxford University Press.

Beckfield, J., Bambra, C., Eikemo, TA., Huijts, T., and Wendt, C. (2015) Towards an institutional theory of welfare state effects on the distribution of population health, *Social Theory and Health*, 13: 227–244.

Biondi M. and Zannino, L. (1997) Psychological stress, neuroimmunomodulation, and susceptibility to infectious diseases in animals and man: A review, *Psychotherapy and Psychosomatics*, 66: 3–26.

Black, D. (1980) Health inequalities: International comparisons, in *Inequalities in Health: The Black Report*, London: Pelican. www.sochealth.co.uk/national-health-service/public-health-and-wellbeing/poverty-and-inequality/the-black-report-1980/black-report-5-health-inequalities-international-comparisons/ [accessed 12/01/21].

Blundell, R., Costa Dias, M., Cribb, J., Joyce, R., Waters, T., Wernham, T., and Xu, X. (2022) Inequality and the COVID-19 crisis in the United Kingdom, *Annual Review of Economics*, 14: 607–636.

Brenner, H. (1995) Political economy and health, in B. Amick and A. Tarlov (eds) *Society and Health*, Oxford: Oxford University Press, pp 211–246.

Buchan, I., Kontopantelis, E., Sperrin, M., Chandola, T., and Doran, T. (2017) North-South disparities in English mortality 1965–2015: Longitudinal population study, *Journal of Epidemiology and Community Health*, 71: 928–936.

Burn, S., Propper, C., Stoye, G., Warner, M., Aylin, P., and Bottle, A. (2021) *What Happened to English NHS Hospital Activity during the COVID-19 Pandemic?*, London: Institute for Fiscal Studies. https://ifs.org.uk/publications/15432 [accessed 15/08/22].

Burstrom, B. and Whitehead, M. (2010) Health inequalities between lone and couple mothers and policy under different welfare regimes: The example of Italy, Sweden and Britain, *Social Science & Medicine*, 70(6): 912–920.

Channing, A., Davies, R., Gabriel, S., Harris, L., Makrelov, K., Robinson, S., Levy, S., Simbanegavi, W., van Seventer, D., and Anderson, L. (2020) COVID-19 lockdowns, income distribution, and food security: An analysis for South Africa, *Global Food Security*, 26: 1000410.

Clair, A. and Hughes, A. (2019) Housing and health: New evidence using biomarker data, *Journal of Epidemiology and Community Health*, 73(3): 256.

Collins, P.H. (2002) *Black Feminist Thought: Knowledge, Consciousness, and the Politics of Empowerment*, New York: Routledge.

Collins, P.H. and Bilge, S. (2016) *Intersectionality*, Cambridge: Policy Press.

Copeland, A., Bambra, C., Nylen, L., Kasim, A.S., Riva, M., Curtis, S., and Burstrom, B. (2013) All in it together? The effects of recession on population health and health inequalities in England and Sweden, 1991 to 2010, *International Journal of Health Services*, 45(45): 3–24.

Corcoran, P., Griffin, E., Arensman, E., Fitzgerald, A.P., and Perry, I.J. (2015) Impact of the economic recession and subsequent austerity on suicide and self-harm in Ireland: An interrupted time series analysis, *International Journal of Epidemiology*, 44: 969–977.

Crenshaw, K. (1989) Demarginalizing the intersection of race and sex: A black feminist critique of anti-discrimination doctrine, feminist theory and antiracist politics, *University of Chicago Legal Forum*, 139: 139–167.

Crenshaw, K. (1991) Mapping the margins: Intersectionality, identity politics, and violence against women of color, *Stanford Law Review*, 1241–1299.

Crenshaw, K. (1992) Whose story is it anyway? Feminist and antiracist appropriations of Anita Hill, in T. Morison (ed) *Race-ing Justice, Engendering Power*, New York: Pantheon.

Crook, H., Raza, S., Nowell, J., Young, M., and Edison, P. (2021) Long COVID: Mechanisms, risk factors, and management, *British Medical Journal*, 374(8303): n1648.

Cummins, S., Curtis, S., Diez-Roux, A., and Macintyre, S. (2007) Understanding and representing 'place' in health research: A relational approach, *Social Science & Medicine*, 65: 1825–1838.

Dahl, E. and Elstad, J.I. (2000) Recent changes in social structure and health inequalities in Norway, *Scandinavian Journal of Public Health. Supplement*, 55: 7–17.

Dahlgren, G. and Whitehead, M. (1991) *Policies and Strategies to Promote Social 9. Equity in Health*, Stockholm: Institute for Future Studies.

Daly, M., Sutin, A.R., and Robinson, E. (2020) Longitudinal changes in mental health and the COVID-19 pandemic: Evidence from the UK Household Longitudinal Study, *Psychological Medicine*, 52(13): 1–10.

Darlington-Pollock, F. and Norman, P. (2017) Examining ethnic inequalities in health and tenure in England: A repeated cross-sectional analysis, *Health & Place*, 46: 82–90.

Darlington-Pollock, F., Norman, P., and Ballas, D. (2017) Using census microdata to explore the inter-relationship between ethnicity, health, socioeconomic factors and internal migration, in J. Stillwell (ed) *The Routledge Handbook of Census Resources, Methods and Applications*, London: Routledge, pp 320–333.

Das-Munshi, J., Bécares, L., Dewey, M.E., Stansfeld, S.A., and Prince, M.J. (2010) Understanding the effect of ethnic density on mental health: multi-level investigation of survey data from England, *British Medical Journal*, 341(7778): c5367.

Davis, A.Y. (1983) *Women, Race and Class*. New York, Vintage Books.

Department for Communities and Local Government (2019) English Indices of Deprivation 2019. https://research.mysociety.org/sites/imd2019/about/ [accessed 22/08/22].

Dorling, D. (2010) 'Persistent North-South Divides', in N. Coe and A. Jones (eds) *The Economic Geography of the UK*, London: Sage Publications.

Dorling, D. (2011) *So You Think You Know about Britain?*, London: Constable.

Economou, M., Madianos, M., Theleritis, C., Peppou, L., and Stefanis, C. (2011) Increased suicidality amid economic crisis in Greece, *Lancet*, 378: 1459.

Eikemo, T. and Bambra, C. (2008) The welfare state: A glossary for public health, *Journal of Epidemiology & Community Health*, 62: 3–6.

Elliott, S.J. (2018) 50 years of medical health geography(ies) of health and wellbeing, *Social Science & Medicine*, 196: 206–208.

Esping-Andersen, G. (1990) *The Three Worlds of Welfare Capitalism*, London: Polity.

Evans, C.R. (2019a) Modelling the intersectionality of processes in the social production of health inequalities, *Social Science & Medicine*, 226: 249–253.

Evans, C.R. (2019b) Reintegrating contexts into quantitative intersectional analyses of health inequalities, *Health & Place*, 60: 102214.

Fagrell Trygg, N., Gustafsson, P.E., and Månsdotter, A. (2019) Languishing in the crossroad? A scoping review of intersectional inequalities in mental health, *International Journal for Equity in Health*, 18: 115.

Fancourt, D., Steptoe, A., and Bu, F. (2021) Trajectories of anxiety and depressive symptoms during enforced isolation due to COVID-19 in England: A longitudinal observational study, *The Lancet Psychiatry*, 8(2): 141–149.

Fox, N.J. and Powell, K. (2021) Place, health and dis/advantage: A sociomaterial analysis, *Health*. doi:10.1177/13634593211014925

Freeman, T., Gesesew, H., Bambra, C., Regina, E., Popay, J., Sanders, D., Macinko, J., Musolino, C., and Baum, F. (2020) Why do some countries do better or worse in life expectancy relative to wealth: An analysis of three countries – Brazil, Ethiopia, and the USA, *International Journal for Equity in Health*, 19: 202.

Gamble, A. (2009) *The Spectre at the Feast: Capitalist Crisis and the Politics of Recession*, Basingstoke: Palgrave.

Gatrell, A. and Elliot, S. (2009) *Geographies of Health: An Introduction*, London: Wiley.

Gerdtham, U. and Ruhm, C. (2006) Deaths rise in good economic times: Evidence from the OECD, *Economics and Human Biology*, 4: 298–316.

Gibson, M., Petticrew, M., Bambra, C., Sowden, A., Wright, K., and Whitehead, J. (2011) Housing and health inequalities: A synthesis of systematic reviews of interventions aimed at different pathways linking housing and health, *Health and Place*, 17: 175–184.

Gili, M., Roca, M., Basu, S., McKee, M., and Stuckler, D. (2013) The mental health risks of economic crisis in Spain: Evidence from primary care centres, 2006 and 2010, *The European Journal of Public Health*, 23(1): 103–108.

Gjonça, A., Brockmann, H. and Maier, H. (2000) Old-age mortality in Germany prior to and after Reunification, *Demographic Research*, 3(1).

Gkiouleka, A, Huijts, T, Beckfield, J., and Bambra, C. (2018) Understanding the Micro and Macro Politics of Health: Inequalities, Intersectionality and Institutions – a research agenda, *Social Science & Medicine*, 200: 92–98.

Goffe, L., Antonopoulouac, V., Meyerac, C., Graham, F., Tangab, M, Lecouturier, J., Grimaniad, A., Bambra, C., Kelly, M., and Sniehotta, F. (2021) Factors associated with vaccine intention in adults living in England who either do not want or have yet decided to be vaccinated against COVID-19, *Human Vaccines & Immunotherapeutics*, 17(12): 2542–2554.

Goodwin, M. and Heath, O. (2016) *Brexit Vote Explained: Poverty, Low Skills and Lack of Opportunities*, York: Joseph Rowntree Foundation. www.jrf.org.uk/report/brexit-vote-explained-poverty-low-skills-and-lack-opportunities [accessed 11/08/2022].

Graham, L., Brown-Jeffy, S., Aronson, R., and Stephens, C. (2011) Critical race theory as theoretical framework and analysis tool for population health research, *Critical Public Health*, 21(1): 81–93.

Guo, L., Wei, D., Zhang, X., Wu, Y., Li, Q., Zhou, M., and Qu, J. (2019) Clinical features predicting mortality risk in patients with viral pneumonia: The MuLBSTA Score, *Front Microbiol.*, 10: 2752.

Hacking, J., Muller, S., and Buchan, I. (2011) Trends in mortality from 1965 to 2008 across the English north–south divide: Comparative observational study, *British Medical Journal*, 342(7794): d508.

Halliday, E., Brennan, L., Bambra, C., and Popay, J. (2021) 'It is surprising how much nonsense you hear': How residents experience and react to living in a stigmatised place – a narrative synthesis of the qualitative evidence, *Health and Place*, 68: 102525.

Halpern, D. and Nazroo, J. (1999) The ethnic density effect: Results from a national community survey of England and Wales, *International Journal of Social Psychiatry*, 46(1): 34–46.

Harvey, D. (2005) *A Brief History of Neoliberalism*, Oxford: Oxford University Press.

Hawe, P. and Shiell, A. (2000) Social capital and health promotion: A review, *Social Science & Medicine*, 51: 871–885.

Hawton, K., Bergen, H., and Geulayov, G. (2016) Impact of the recent recession on self-harm: A longitudinal ecologic and patient level investigation from multicentre study of self-harm in England, *Journal of Affective Disorders*, 191: 132–138.

Holdroyd, I., Vodden, A., Srinivasan, A., Kuhn, I., Bambra, C., and Ford, J. (2022) Systematic review of the effectiveness of the health inequalities strategy in England between 1999 and 2010, *British Medical Journal*, 12(9): e063137.

Holman, D., Bell, A., Green, M., and Salway, S. (2022) Neighbourhood deprivation and intersectional inequalities in biomarkers of healthy ageing in England, *Health & Place*, 77: 102871.

Holt, D. (1999) Overview of the Medicare and Medicaid programs, Health Care Financing Review, Spring 1999.

hooks, b. (1981) *Ain't I a Woman Black Women and Feminism*, Cambridge: South End Press.

Hopkins, P. (2018) Feminist geographies and intersectionality, *Gender, Place & Culture*, 25(4): 585–590.

Hopkins, P. (2019) Social geography I: Intersectionality, *Progress in Human Geography*, 43: 937–947.

Hopkins, P., Botterill, K., Sanghera, G., and Arshad, R. (2017) Encountering misrecognition: Being mistaken for being Muslim, *Annals of the American Association of Geographers*, 107(4): 934–948.

Houdmont, J., Kerr, R., and Addley, K. (2012) Psychosocial factors and economic recession: The Stormont Study, *Occupational Medicine*, 62(2): 98–104.

Iyer, A., Sen, G., and Ostlin, P. (2008) The intersections of gender and class in health status and health care, *Global Public Health*, 3(S1): 13–24.

Kapilashrami, A., Hill, S., and Meer, N. (2015) What can health inequalities researchers learn from an intersectionality perspective? Understanding social dynamics with an inter-categorical approach?, *Soc Theory Health*, 13: 288–307.

Karger, H. and Stoesz, D. (1990) *American Social Welfare Policy*, New York: Longman.

Katikireddi, S.V., Niedzwiedz, C.L., and Popham, F. (2012) Trends in population mental health before and after the 2008 recession: A repeat cross-sectional analysis of the 1991–2010 Health Surveys of England, *British Medical Journal*, 2(5).

Katikireddi, S.V., Lal, S., Carrol, E.D., Niedzwiedz, C.L., Khunti, K., Dundas, R. et al (2021) Unequal impact of the COVID-19 crisis on minority ethnic groups: A framework for understanding and addressing inequalities, *Journal of Epidemiology and Community Health*, 75(10): 970–974.

Kondo, N., Subramanian, S., Kawachi, I., Takeda, Y., and Yamagata, Z. (2008) Economic recession and health inequalities in Japan: Analysis with a national sample, 1986–2001, *Journal of Epidemiology and Community Health*, 62: 869–875.

Krieger, N. (1997) Measuring social class in US public health research: Concepts, methodologies and guidelines, *Annual Review of Public Health*, 18(1): 341–378.

Krieger, N. (2000) Discrimination and health, *Social Epidemiology*, 1: 36–75.

Krieger N. (2003) Theories for social epidemiology in the twenty-first century: An ecosocial perspective, in R. Hofrichter (ed) *Health and Social Justice: Politics, Ideology, and Inequity in the Distribution of Disease – a Public Health Reader*, San Francisco: Jossey-Bass, pp 428–450.

Krieger, N., Rehkopf, D., Chen, J, Waterman, P., Marcelli, E., and Kennedy, M. (2008) The fall and rise of US inequities in premature mortality: 1960–2002, *PLoS Medicine*, 5: 227–241.

Krieger, N., Chen, J., Coull, B., Waterman, P., and Beckfield, J. (2013) The unique impact of abolition of Jim Crow laws on reducing inequities in infant death rates and implications for choice of comparison groups in analyzing societal determinants of health, *American Journal of Public Health*, 103: 2234–44.

Krieger, N., Chen, J., Coull, B., Beckfield, J., Kiang, M., and Waterman, P. (2014) Jim Crow and premature mortality among the US Black and White population, 1960–2009: An age-period-cohort analysis, *Epidemiology*, 25: 494–504.

Krieger, N., Jahn, J., and Waterman, P. (2017) Jim Crow and estrogen-receptor-negative breast cancer: US-born black and white non-Hispanic women, 1992–2012, *Cancer Causes Control*, 28: 49–59.

Lacobucci, G. (2019) GPs in deprived areas face severest pressures, *British Medical Journal*, 365: l2104.

Lahelma, E., Kivelä, K., Roos, E., Tuominen, T., Dahl, E., Diderichsen, F., and Yngwe, M.Å. (2002) Analysing changes of health inequalities in the Nordic welfare states, *Social Science & Medicine*, 55(4): 609–625.

Landmann Szwarcwald, C., da Silva de Almeida, W., Azeredo Teixeira, R., Barboza França, E., Jorge de Miranda, M., and Carvalho Malta, D. (2020) Inequalities in infant mortality in Brazil at subnational levels in Brazil, 1990 to 2015, *Popul. Health Metrics*, 18: 4.

Lassale, C., Gaye, B., Hamer, M., Gale, C.R., and Batty, G.D. (2020) Ethnic disparities in hospitalisation for COVID-19 in England: the role of socioeconomic factors, mental health, and inflammatory and pro-inflammatory factors in a community-based cohort study, *Brain, Behavior, and Immunity*, 88: 44–49.

Lundberg, O. (1986) Class and health: Comparing Britain and Sweden, *Soc Sci Med.*, 26: 511–517.

Lundberg, O. and E. Lahelma (2001) Nordic health inequalities in the European context, in M. Kautto, J. Fritzell, B. Hvinden, J. Kvist and H. Uusitalo (eds) *Nordic Welfare States in the European Context*, London: Routledge, pp 42–65.

Lundberg, O., Diderichsen, F., and Yngwe, M. Å. (2001) Changing health inequalities in a changing society? Sweden in the mid-1980s and mid-1990s, *Scandinavian Journal of Public Health*, 29: 31–39.

Macinko, J., Guanais, F., and De Souza, M. (2006) An evaluation of the impact of the Family Health Program on infant mortality in Brazil 1990–2002, *Journal of Epidemiology and Community Health*, 60(1): 13–19.

Macintyre, S. (2007) Deprivation amplification revisited: Or, is it always true that poorer places have poorer access to resources for healthy diets and physical activity?, *International Journal of Behavioral Nutrition and Physical Activity*, 43: 1–7.

Macintyre, S., Maciver, S., and Sooman, A. (1993) Area, class and health: Should we be focusing on places or people?, *Journal of Social Policy*, 22: 213–234.

Macintyre, S., Ellaway, A., and Cummins, S. (2002) Place effects on health: How can we conceptualise, operationalise and measure them?, *Social Science & Medicine*, 55(1): 125–139.

Macintyre, S., Macdonald, L., and Ellaway, A. (2008) Do poorer people have poorer access to local resources and facilities? The distribution of local resources by area deprivation in Glasgow, Scotland, *Social Science & Medicine*, 67: 900e14.

Manderbacka, K., Lahelma, E., and Rahkonen, O. (2001) Structural changes and social inequalities in health in Finland, 1986–1994, *Scandinavian Journal of Public Health*, 29: 41–54.

Marmot, M. (2020) The Marmot Review: Ten years on, The Health Foundation. www.health.org.uk/publications/reports/the-mar mot-review-10-years-on [accessed 08/08/22].

McGowan, V. and Bambra, C. (2022) COVID-19 mortality and deprivation: Pandemic, syndemic and endemic health inequalities, *Lancet Public Health*, 7(11): E966–E975.

McNamara, C., Balaj, M., Thomson, K., Eikemo, T., and Bambra, C. (2017) The contribution of housing and neighbourhood conditions to educational inequalities in non-communicable diseases in Europe: Findings from the European Social Survey (2014) special module on the social determinants of health, *European Journal of Public Health*, 27 (suppl_1): 102–106.

Monteiro, C., Benicio, M., Konno, S., Silva, A., Lima, A., and Conde, W. (2009) Cause for the decline in child undernutrition in Brazil, 1996–2007, *Rev Saude Publica*, 43: 35–43.

Montgomery, S., Cook, D., Bartley, M., and Wadsworth, M. (1999a) Unemployment pre-dates symptoms of depression and anxiety resulting in medical consultation in young men, *International Journal of Epidemiology*, 28: 95–100.

Montgomery, S., Cook, D., Bartley, M., and Wadsworth, M. (1999b) Unemployment, cigarette smoking, alcohol consumption and body weight in young British men, *European Journal of Public Health*, 8: 21–27.

Munford, L., Khavandi, S., Bambra, C., Barr, B., Davies, H., Doran, T., Kontopantelis, E., Norman, P., Pickett, K., Sutton, M., and Taylor-Robinson, D. (2021) *A Year of COVID-19 in the North: Regional Inequalities in Health and Economic Outcomes*, Newcastle: NHSA. www.thenhsa.co.uk/app/uploads/2021/09/A-Year-of-COVID-in-the-North-report-2021.pdf [accessed 08/08/22].

Munford, L., Khavandi, S., and Bambra, C. (2022a) COVID-19 and Deprivation Amplification: An Ecological Study of Geographical Inequalities in Mortality in England, *Health Place*, November.

Munford, L., Mott, L., Davies, H., McGowan, V., and Bambra, C. (2022b) Overcoming health inequalities in 'left behind' neighbourhoods, Northern Health Science Alliance and the APPG for 'left behind' neighbourhoods. www.appg-leftbehindneighbourhoods.org.uk/wp-content/uploads/2022/01/Overcoming-Health-Inequalities.pdf [accessed 17/08/22].

Nandi, A. and Platt, L. (2020) Briefing note COVID-19 survey: ethnic differences in effects of COVID-19: household and local context, Briefing note. www.understandingsociety.ac.uk/research/publications/526259 [accessed 11/10/2022].

Nash, J.C. (2008) Re-thinking intersectionality, *Feminist Review*, 89(1): 1–15.

National Institute for Health and Care Excellence (2020) COVID-19 rapid guideline: Managing the long-term effects of COVID-19 NICE guideline. www.nice.org.uk/guidance/ng188

Nazroo, J.Y. and Bécares, L. (2020) Evidence for ethnic inequalities in mortality related to COVID-19 infections: Findings from an ecological analysis of England, *British Medical Journal*, 10(12): 041750.

Nazroo, J.Y. and Williams, D.R. (2005) The social determination of ethnic/racial inequalities in health, *Social Determinants of Health*, 2: 238–266.

Nguyen, L.H., Drew, D.A., Graham, M.S., Joshi, A.D., Guo, C.G., Ma, W., Mehta, R.S., Warner, E.T., Sikavi, D.R., Lo, C.H., and Kwon, S. (2020) Risk of COVID-19 among front-line health-care workers and the general community: A prospective cohort study, *The Lancet Public Health*, 5(9): e475–e483.

NHS Digital (2021) Coronavirus shielded patient list summary totals, England. https://digital.nhs.uk/data-and-information/publications/statistical/mi-english-coronavirus-covid-19-shielded-patient-list-summary-totals [accessed 22/08/22].

Niedzwiedz, C.L. Mitchell, R.J. Shortt, N.K., and Pearce, J.R. (2016) Social protection spending and inequalities in depressive symptoms across Europe, *Social Psychiatry and Psychiatric Epidemiology*, 51(7): 1005–1014.

Niedzwiedz, C.L., Green, M.J., Benzeval, M., Campbell, D., Craig, P., Demou, E. et al (2021) Mental health and health behaviours before and during the initial phase of the COVID-19 lockdown: Longitudinal analyses of the UK Household Longitudinal Study, *Journal of Epidemiology and Community Health*, 75(3): 224–231.

Nolte, E., Brand, A., Koupilová, I., and McKee, M. (2000) Neonatal and postneonatal mortality in Germany since unification, *Journal of Epidemiology and Community Health*, 54: 84–90.

Nolte, E., Scholz, R., Shkolnikov, V., and McKee, M. (2002) The contribution of medical care to changing life expectancy in Germany and Poland, *Social Science & Medicine*, 55: 1905–1921.

O'Connor, R.C., Wetherall, K., Cleare, S., McClelland, H., Melson, A.J., Niedzwiedz, C.L., O'Carroll, R.E., O'Connor, D.B., Platt, S., Scowcroft, E., and Watson, B. (2021) Mental health and well-being during the COVID-19 pandemic: longitudinal analyses of adults in the UK COVID-19 Mental Health & Wellbeing study, *The British Journal of Psychiatry*, 218(6): 326–333.

Office for National Statistics (2016) Output areas. www.ons.gov.uk/census/2001censusandearlier/dataandproducts/outputgeography/outputareas [accessed 22/08/22].

Office for National Statistics. (2021) Coronavirus and depression in adults, Great Britain: January to March 2021. www.ons.gov.uk/releases/coronavirusanddepressioninadultsgreatbritainjanuarytomarch2021 [accessed: 10/03/22].

Office for National Statistics (2022) Prevalence of ongoing Symptoms following coronavirus (COVID-19) infection in the UK. www.ons.gov.uk/peoplepopulationandcommunity/healthandsocialcare/conditionsanddiseases/datasets/alldatarelatingtoprevalenceofongoingsymptomsfollowingcoronaviruscovid19infectionintheuk [accessed 20/06/22].

Packard, J. (2003) *American Nightmare: The History of Jim Crow*, New York: St Martin's Press.

Pearce, J., Blakely, T., Witten, K., and Bartie, P. (2007) Neighborhood deprivation and access to fast-food retailing – A national study, *American Journal of Preventive Medicine*, 32: 375–382.

Petersen, C.B., Mortensen, L.H., Morgen, C.S., Madsen, M., Schnor, o., Arntzen, A., Gissler, M., Cnattingius, S., and Nybo Andersen., A. (2009) Socio-economic inequality in preterm birth: A comparative study of the Nordic countries from 1981 to 2000, *Paediatric and Perinatal Epidemiology*, 23(1): 66–75.

Pierce, M., Hope, H., Ford, T., Hatch, S., Hotopf, M., John, A., Kontopantelis, E., Webb, R., Wessely, S., McManus, S., and Abel, K.M. (2020) Mental health before and during the COVID-19 pandemic: A longitudinal probability sample survey of the UK population, *The Lancet Psychiatry*, 7(10): 883–892.

Powell, K., Barnes, A., Anderson de Cuevas, R., Bambra, C., Halliday, E., Lewis, S. et al (2020) Power, control, communities and health inequalities III: Participatory spaces: An English case, Health Promotion International. doi: 10.1093/heapro/daaa059

Proto, E. and Quintana-Domeque, C. (2021) COVID-19 and mental health deterioration by ethnicity and gender in the UK, *PLoS ONE*, 16(1): e0244419.

Public Health England (2013) Longer lives. http://longerlives.phe.org.uk/ [accessed 08/08/22].

Public Health England (2020a) Fingertips dashboard. https://fingertips.phe.org.uk/ [accessed 08/08/22].

Public Health England (2020b) Disparities in the risk and outcomes of COVID-19, Public Health England.

Ritakallio, V.M. and Fritzell, J. (2004) Societal Shifts and Changed Patterns of Poverty, *Luxembourg Income Study Working Paper Series*.

Robinson, T., Brown, H., Norman, P., Barr, B., Fraser, L., and Bambra, C. (2019) Investigating the impact of New Labour's English health inequalities strategy on geographical inequalities in infant mortality: a time trend analysis, *Journal of Epidemiology and Community Health*, 73: 564–568.

Rocha, V., Ribero, I., Severo, M., Barros, H., and Fraga, S. (2017) Neighbourhood socioeconomic deprivation and health-related quality of life: A multilevel analysis, *PLoS ONE*, 12(12): e0188736.

Rodo´-de-Zarate, M. (2014) Developing geographies of intersectionality with relief maps: Reflections from youth research in Manresa, *Catalonia. Gender, Place and Culture*, 21: 925–944.

Roncon, L., Zuin, M., Rigatelli, G., and Zuliani, G. (2020) Diabetic patients with COVID-19 infection are at higher risk of ICU admission and poor short-term outcome, *Journal of Clinical Virology*, 127: 104354.

Ruhm, C.J. (2000) Are recessions good for your health?, *Quarterly Journal of Economics*, 115(2): 617–650.

Russell, D. (2004) *Looking North: Northern England and the National Imagination*, Manchester, Manchester University Press.

Rutter, P., Mytton, O., Mak, M., and Donaldson, L. (2012) Socio-economic disparities in mortality due to pandemic influenza in England, *International Journal of Public Health*, 57: 745–750.

Saez, E. and Zucman, G. (2014) Wealth inequality in the United States since 1913: Evidence from capitalized income tax data, in NBER Working Paper, N.B.o.E. Research, Editor. Cambridge, National Bureau of Economic Research.

Saunders, R., Buckman, J.E., Fonagy, P., and Fancourt, D. (2021) Understanding different trajectories of mental health across the general population during the COVID-19 pandemic, *Psychological Medicine*, 1–9.

Schneider, S., Bolbos, A., Fessler, J., and Buck, C. (2019) Deprivation amplification due to structural disadvantage? Playgrounds as important physical activity resources for children and adolescents, *Public Health*, 168: 117–127.

Schrecker, T. and Bambra., C. (2015) *How Politics Makes Us Sick: Neoliberal Epidemics*, London, Palgrave Macmillan.

Schroeder, C.G. (2014) (Un)holy Toledo: Intersectionality, interdependence, and neighbourhood (trans)formation in Toledo, Ohio, *Annals of the Association of American Geographers*, 104: 166–181.

Scott-Samuel, A., Bambra, C., Collins, C., Hunter, D.J., McCartney, G., and Smith, K. (2014) The impact of Thatcherism on health and wellbeing in Britain, *International Journal of Health Services*, 44: 53–72.

Scruggs, L., Detlef, J., and Kuitto, K. (2014) *Comparative Welfare Entitlements Dataset 2, Version 2014–03*, Mansfield: University of Connecticut.

Segerstrom, S.C. and Miller, G.E. (2004) Psychological stress and the human immune system: A meta-analytic study of 30 years of inquiry, *Psychol Bull*, 4: 601–630.

Shaw, C., Blakely, T., Atkinson, J., and Crampton, P. (2005) Do social and economic reforms change socioeconomic inequalities in child mortality? A case study: New Zealand 1981–1999, *Journal of Epidemiology and Community Health*, 59(8): 638–644.

Simonnet, A., Chetboun, M., Poissy, J., Raverdy, V., Noulette, J., Duhamel, A., Labreuche, J., Mathieu, D., Pattou, F., and Jourdain, M. (2020) High prevalence of obesity in severe acute respiratory syndrome coronavirus-2 (SARS-CoV-2) requiring invasive mechanical ventilation, *Obesity*. doi:10.1002/ oby.22831

Simpson, J., Albani, V., Bell, Z., Bambra, C., and Brown, H. (2021) Effects of social security policy reforms on mental health and inequalities: A systematic review of observational studies in high-income countries, *Social Science & Medicine*, 272: 113717.

Singer M. (2000) A dose of drugs, a touch of violence, a case of AIDS: Conceptualizing the SAVA syndemic, *Free Inq Creat Sociol*, 28: 13–24.

Singer, M. (2009) *Introduction to Syndemics: A Systems Approach to Public and Community Health*, San Francisco, CA: Jossey-Bass.

Skalická, V., Lenthe, F., Bambra, C., Krokstad, S., and Mackenbach J. (2009) Material, psychosocial, behavioural and biomedical factors in the explanation of socio-economic inequalities in mortality: Evidence from the HUNT study, *International Journal of Epidemiology*, 38: 1272–1284.

Smith, G., Chaturvedi, N., Harding, S., Nazroo, J., and Williams, R. (2003) Ethnic inequalities in health: A review of UK epidemiological evidence, in G.D. Smith (ed) *Health Inequalities: Lifecourse Approaches*, Bristol: Policy Press, pp 271–309.

Smith, K.E., Hill, S., and Bambra, C. (eds) (2016) *Health Inequalities: Critical Perspectives*, Oxford: Oxford University Press.

Tapia Granados, J.A. (2005) Increasing mortality during the expansions of the US economy, 1900–1996, *International Journal of Epidemiology*, 34: 1194–1202.

Taylor-Robinson, D., Lai, E., Wickham, S., Rose, T., Bambra, C., Whitehead, M., and Barr, B. (2019) Assessing the impact of rising child poverty on the unprecedented rise in infant mortality in England, 2000–2017: Time trend analysis, *British Medical Journal*, 9: e029424.

Thompson, L., Pearce, J., and Barnett, R. (2007) Moralising geographies: Stigma, smoking islands and responsible subjects, *Area*, 39: 508–517.

Todd, A. and Bambra, C. (2021) Learning from past mistakes? The COVID-19 Vaccine and the Inverse Equity Hypothesis, *European Journal of Public Health*, 31: 2.

Todd, A., Copeland, A., Husband, A., Kasim, A., and Bambra, C. (2015) Access all areas? An area-level analysis of the relationship between community pharmacy and primary care distribution, urbanity and social deprivation in England, *British Medical Journal*, 5: e007328.

Vagero, D. and Lundberg, O. (1989) Health inequalities in Britain and Sweden, *Lancet*, ii: 35–36.

Valkonen, T. (1989) *Adult Mortality and Level of Education: A Comparison of Six Countries. Health Inequalities in European Countries*, ed A.J. Fox, Aldershot, Gower, pp 142–160.

Valkonen, T., Martikainen, P., Jalovaara, M., Koskinen, S., Martelin, T., and Makela, P. (2000) Changes in socioeconomic inequalities in mortality during an economic boom and recession among middle-aged men and women in Finland, *European Journal of Public Health*, 10: 274–80.

Victora, C., Aquino, E., do Carmo Leal, M., Monteiro, C., Barros, F., and Szwarcwald, C. (2011) Maternal and child health in Brazil: Progress and challenges, *Lancet*, 377: 1863–1876.

Vizard, P. and Obolenskaya, P. (2015) The Coalition's Record on Health: Policy, Spending and Outcomes 2010–2015. Social Policy in a Cold Climate Working Paper, 16.

Walton, H., Dajnak, D., Beevers, S., Williams, M., Watkiss, P., and Hunt, A. (2015) *Understanding the Health Impacts of Air Pollution in London*, London: Kings College. https://data.london.gov.uk/download/5fbda6f4-06a9-4b50-99e6-ef6507018c2e/ea00c246-da42-4335-a01f-60c5b7fc0df7/HIAinLondon_KingsReport_14072015_final.pdf [accessed 08/08/22].

Ward, K. and England, K. (2007) *Introduction: Reading Neoliberalization*, in K. England and K. Ward, eds, *Neoliberalization: States, Networks, People*, Blackwell: Oxford.

Weber, L. and Parra-Medina, D. (2003) Intersectionality and women's health: Charting a path to eliminating health disparities, *Advances in Gender Research*, 7: 181–230.

Welsh, C., Albani, V., Matthews, F., and Bambra, C. (2022) Inequalities in the evolution of the COVID-19 pandemic: An ecological study of inequalities in mortality in the first wave and the effects of the first national lockdown in England, *British Medical Journal*, 12: e058658.

Whitehead, M. and Popay, J. (2010) Swimming upstream? Taking action on the social determinants of health inequalities, *Social Science & Medicine*, 71: 1234–1236.

Whitehead, M., Bambra, C., Barr, B., Bowles, J., Caulfield, R., Doran, T., Harrison, D., Lynch, A., Pleasant, S., and Weldon, J. (2014) *Due North: Report of the Inquiry on Health Equity for the North*, Liverpool: University of Liverpool and Centre for Local Economic Strategies. https://cles.org.uk/wp-content/uploads/2016/11/Due-North-Report-of-the-Inquiry-on-Health-Equity-in-the-North-final.pdf [accessed 08/08/22].

Whitehead, M., Pennington, A., Orton, L., Nayak, S., Petticrew, M., Sowden, A., and White, M. (2016) How could differences in 'control over destiny' lead to socio-economic inequalities in health? A synthesis of theories and pathways in the living environment, *Health and Place*, 39: 51–61.

WHO (World Health Organization) (2008) Closing the gap in a generation: Health equity through action on the social determinants of health, Geneva: World Health Organization. www.who.int/social_determinants/thecommission/finalreport/en/ [accessed 08/08/22].

WHO (World Health Organization) (2022) *Tobacco Factsheet*. www.who.int/news-room/fact-sheets/detail/tobacco [accessed 08/08/22].

Yuval-Davis, N. (2015) Situated intersectionality and social inequality, *Raisons politiques*, 58(2): 91–100.

Zavras, D., Tsiantou, V., Pavi, E., Mylona, K., and Kyriopoulos, J. (2013) Impact of economic crisis and other demographic and socio-economic factors on self-rated health in Greece, *The European Journal of Public Health*, 23(2): 206–210.

Index

References to figures appear in *italic* type; those in **bold** type refer to tables. References to endnotes show both the page number and the note number (111n7).